6 Steps to Understanding and Coping with Mild Traumatic Brain Injury

Strategies to dealing with Cognitive Function Loss, Self Esteem, Relationships and Fatigue

By Jade Roberts

This book expresses the author's personal courage and determination in her path to recovery. The book is an example of what people need in the way of motivation for recovery. The author demonstrates how victims can take their injury as a personal challenge. The author's personal recovery was only made possible because defeat was never accepted or surrendered to. The author is a shining real-life example for others facing recovery from brain trauma. This book is so important since it inspires people to try and try harder and never give up. We don't have a choice to have or not have a brain injury. We do have a choice what we do about it, and how we feel about it. This book means to inspire hope, encourage the power of determination and strong will as a key component to successful brain injury rehabilitation. The power of personal outlook and optimism is as important as medication, occupational therapy, talking therapies or any other help.

Dr Peter M Berger, Ed.D., CPsychol / MBACP

****

This book confronts MTBI head on, with a realistic, truthful and heartfelt approach.

It gives the reader a well-rounded appraisal of the condition, with its many forms, in an easy to read manner to which you don't need a medical background to understand. Most importantly, its breaks down the barriers the sufferer may have, to getting the help they need.

Caroline Gilroy, Chiropractor

Foreword

This book was developed as a result of my own experience as an MTBI sufferer (Mild Traumatic Brain Injury). It was two years after the injury, before I could get an accurate diagnosis of my problems, and three years before effective therapies began to change my life for the better.

Due to the lack of readily available information, I did not understand what had happened to me. I was frustrated and traumatized which made my recovery more difficult.

I hope this book will fill that gap for others like me and will aid them in finding the help they need; as well as beginning the journey of understanding and accepting the ways MTBI has changed their lives.

A book about brain trauma of any kind is ambitious in and of itself. This, however, is a book about mild traumatic brain injury, a problem of epidemic but largely silent proportions that is only now beginning to be understood by both medical science and the general public.

Injuries like those suffered in 2006 in Iraq by ABC News anchorman Bob Woodruff and in 2011 in Tucson by Arizona Congresswoman Gabrielle Giffords grab headlines. Yet the vast majority of brain injuries – as many as 90% - are concussions that occur under far more humble circumstances.

The most common causes are falls, traffic accidents, struck by and against events like those that happen in contact sports, and assaults. Add to that mild brain injuries caused by some degree of oxygen deprivation. It's not difficult to understand how 1.7 million people in the U.S. and 1 million in Europe are the victims of MTBI annually.

Injuries from lack of oxygen occur most typically from carbon monoxide poisoning, drowning, choking, suffocation, head trauma, severe bleeding, drops in blood pressure, stroke, and anaesthesia/surgical errors.

But concussion is the primary culprit, an injury in which the motion and impact of the brain within the skull leads to the straining, stretching and even tearing of axons or nerve cells.

One concussion is sufficient to alter brain function for life. Serial concussions are now linked to severe early onset dementia in retired NFL athletes (American National Football League).

Traditionally a concussion has been seen as something you just shake off. Most people don't lose consciousness, and it may be hours or even days before symptoms surface. There have been no good tests for the presence of concussion and in fact most people who suffer from MTBI tend not to seek treatment unless it's absolutely necessary. They're terrified by what they're experiencing, and they don't want anyone else to find out, usually for fear of their jobs being in peril.

In Europe, however, blood tests to detect the presence of the protein S100B are standard to determine if a concussion has occurred. The protein exists only in the brain. If it's present in the bloodstream, the blood/brain barrier has been compromised.

Until such a test is considered standard globally, however, people with brain injuries are being sent back to work – or worse yet back on the sports playing field – with no proper recognition of just how badly hurt they may be.

Brain injury is unique to the individual, but there are common denominators present in every case. The first step in bringing MTBI out of the shadows is education, both for the person suffering the injury and for their friends and loved ones.

The purpose of this book is to lay a foundation for that education. I am not a doctor and this is not meant to be an exhaustive medical discussion of MTBI. At the end of this book, however, you should be able to ask better questions and seek better answers than those that are currently being provided to MTBI sufferers, including the most frightening one of all. "Go home and rest for a couple of days." If only it was always that simple!

Acknowledgements

To the medical professionals Dr Gillian Levett, Dr Udo Kischka and Dr Greenwood who finally put my spiritual self at ease when they explained I had sustained hypoxic brain injury.

To Dr Alner and Dr Hemberger who worked with me to identify the areas of my cognitive functioning which were affected and helped me to put in place strategies to make my life more manageable.

Dr Peter Berger my CBT therapist who devoted time to make me accept the "new" me and also encouraged me to build my relationships around me again.

My husband Stephen and daughter Amy who have given me unconditional support and love through the difficult times and the good times.

To my Mum, late Dad and all my siblings for their devoted love and support for which I will always be indebted.

To everyone who has touched my life over the years, and have been a great pillar of support, friendship and comradeship.

Table of Contents

Chapter 1 - Introduction to Minimal and Brain Trauma

This is not a book about severe brain trauma or about the often devastating physical disabilities that are caused by such injuries. This book is about a largely silent epidemic.

Studies estimate that 75% to 90% of all traumatic brain injuries are concussions or some other form of MTBI — mild traumatic brain injury — a form of neurological wound is often discounted or downplayed even by the person suffering from the injury.

What the Media Reports about Brain Injury

Since 2002, the wars in Iraq and Afghanistan have placed traumatic brain injury firmly in the forefront of news reports. This was particularly true after ABC News anchorman Bob Woodruff was almost killed by a roadside bomb near Taji, Iraq in 2006.

In a stunning recovery, largely reflective of what military doctors in the field learned first-hand about treating brain injuries, Woodruff returned to work 13 months later.

Woodruff's journey started with a 36-day medically induced coma. He then went through nine surgeries to remove parts of his skull and to control the pressure being placed on his brain.

Although his physical abilities returned with remarkable speed, his cognitive rehabilitation was intense. Seven years later Woodruff still struggles with language difficulties, blindness in the upper quarter of both eyes, and hearing loss.

Woodruff's recovery, and that of Arizona Congresswoman Gabrielle Giffords who was shot in Tucson in 2011, are dramatic and inspiring. However, outcomes like that experienced by Andrew Blackmore-Dobbyn are more typical.

For Blackmore-Dobbyn, and for the vast number of brain injury survivors of limited financial means, the expensive and lengthy treatments often necessary for a full recovery simply are not possible. For people in the United States with no health insurance, there is not even a hope for that level of treatment.

In the United Kingdom, with the National Health Service, possible delays in diagnoses and treatment are common.

Blackmore-Dobbyn, a New York chef, was attacked on the street and punched repeatedly in the face, choked, and had his head slammed into the sidewalk. Any of these traumas would have been sufficient to cause MTBI.

In an article for The Huffington Post in November 2011, "Why Gabby Giffords' Recovery Is Not a Miracle," Blackmore-Dobbyn made it clear that he does not begrudge the level of care the congresswoman was fortunate enough to receive.

Blackmore-Dobbyn, however, lost his job, and had no one on whom to rely for care but his wife. *"I no longer function at the same level due to chronic anxiety, permanent short-term memory impairment and a diminished capacity for multi-tasking, all of which are so vitally important in the work of a restaurant kitchen,"* he wrote.

"I now work in a lesser capacity and will earn less money during my lifetime as a result. In short, I was financially, professionally, and emotionally ruined. I don't know if it would have been different

if I'd had access to a team of rehabilitation specialists. I wish that I'd had the option."

Blackmore-Dobbyn was physically assaulted, but he could have just as easily been in an automobile accident, fallen off a ladder, or been injured repeatedly playing contact sports and experienced similar long-term consequences. This is what the vast majority of people do not understand about the meaning of **"mild"** traumatic brain injury.

Where MTBI is Concerned, Language is Deceiving

Words can be misleading. In reference to brain injury, terms like "minimal", "moderate", or "mild" are widely misconstrued. The initial trauma may be "mild." The person may not lose consciousness, and there may be no apparent symptoms or deficits for hours or even days. That's the insidious nature of this level of brain trauma.

There is likely nothing "mild" about the consequences of the injury, however. In fact, one of the major hurdles in diagnosing MTBI lies in the reaction of the patients themselves.

Whether they are in denial about the presence of the injury, or aware of it and hiding their problems out of fear of rejection, loss, or criticism, it's much more common for MTBI sufferers to NOT seek treatment. It may also be that the individual does not think a brain injury is a possibility. They simply know that something isn't right. In any of these cases the person tries to cope on their own even to the point of self-isolation or self-medication.

They know they are having headaches and trouble concentrating, that they get anxious or irritable, or can't stand bright lights and loud noises, but they don't look injured. Maybe they just "got their bell rung" playing football or were involved in a fender bender. That's just something you shake off, right? Wrong.

How is MTBI diagnosed?

Accurately diagnosing MTBI is a major hurdle standing in the way of proper treatment. The criteria developed by the Centres for Disease Control in the United States are as follows:

- An injury to the head from blunt force, acceleration, or deceleration.

One or more of the following must then be present immediately after the event or during a period of observation.

- Observed or self-reported impaired consciousness, disorientation, or transient confusion.

- Observed or self-reported amnesia around the time of the injury.

- Observed signs of neuropsychological or neurological dysfunction.

These symptoms may include, but are not limited to:

- seizures

- irritability, lethargy, vomiting (especially in infants and very young children)

- headaches, dizziness, fatigue, poor concentration (in older children and adults)

14

The CDC definition, however, requires "loss of consciousness or altered consciousness" lasting 30 minutes or less for these symptoms to point to MTBI.

The Brain Injury Association of America in its website materials on "Mild Brain Injury and Concussion" takes exception with this approach, writing:

"The definition focuses on the actual injury or symptoms, not the possible consequences. For many people, there are challenges in getting an accurate diagnosis and treatment, especially when there is no documented or observed loss of consciousness. There does not need to be a loss of consciousness for a brain injury to occur."

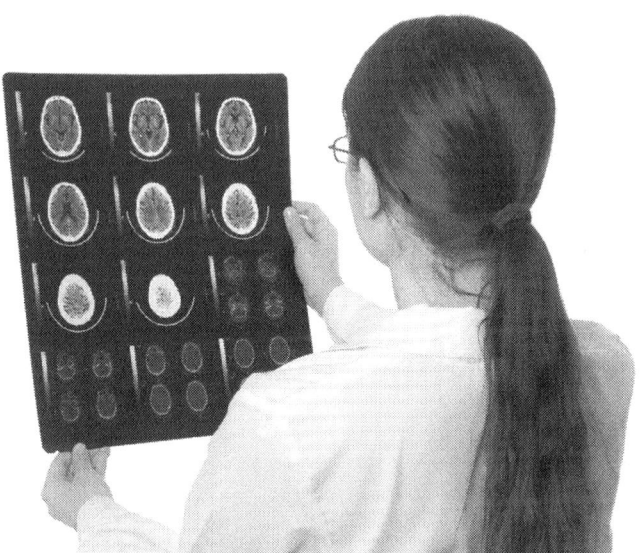

The issue of accurate diagnoses will be discussed at greater length in Chapter 3 - Diagnosing Minimal and Moderate Brain Trauma, but this is definitely an area of MTBI treatment that is still in need of refinement and vigilant application.

The Definition of MTBI and Its Major Causes

The definition of MTBI is more precise than the diagnostic criteria. Due to an external force that is either accidental or deliberate, an alteration in brain function occurs. This may be from a direct blow, a "blast" force, or the rapid acceleration or deceleration of the head.

A penetrating injury is not present, and there may be no loss of consciousness. The true extent of the damage will not be readily apparent and will develop over time.

The leading causes of MTBI in the United States:

- falls 35.2% (in the U.S.)

Falls account for half of brain injuries in children age 0-14, and 61% among adults age 65 and above.

- motor vehicle / traffic accidents 17%

- struck by / against events 16.5%

These events include colliding with a stationary or a moving object, and represent the second leading cause of brain injury among children 0-14 (in 25% of cases.)

- assaults 10%

Assaults account for 2.9% of brain injuries in children 0-14, and 1% of cases in adults 65 and older.

- other 21%

In the United States, 18% of brain injuries occur in children 0-4, with approximately 22% of cases in adults 75 and older. In 59% of cases, the patients are males.

Approximately 1.7 million people in the U.S. suffer some type of brain injury annually. Of those, more than 475,000 are children.

Each year, more than 50,000 people die as the result of brain trauma.

It is estimated that 3.1 million American citizens live with a lifetime disability related to a brain injury.

The CDC calculates the medical costs and lost productivity per year to brain injury in excess of $76.3 billion.

(**See**: "What Are the Leading Causes of TBI?" The Centers for Disease Control http://www.cdc.gov/traumaticbraininjury/causes.html Accessed June 2013.)

In Europe, the leading causes of MTBI are:

- motor vehicle crashes, 50%

This figure is inclusive of autos, trucks, motorcycles, bicycles, and pedestrian injuries.

- falls, in the 65+ age range

- transportation injuries in the age 65 and under age range

- sports-related injuries (300,000 annually)

Of those, some 20,000 are caused by skiing, ice-skating, and other winter sports.

There are approximately 1 million head injuries per year in Europe, with some 135,000 patients admitted to hospital for treatment.

It is estimated that across Europe there are 500,000 people age 16-74 living with long-term disabilities due to brain injury.

Of the annual reported injuries, 85% are classified as minor.

Men are 2-3 times more likely to suffer a brain injury, with those aged 15-20 five times more likely.

(**See**: "Brain Injury Facts," International Brain Injury Association, http://www.internationalbrain.org/brain-injury-facts/ - Accessed June 2013.)

Difficulty in Detecting MTBI

Brain injuries are classified as focal or diffuse. A focal brain injury occurs in a precise location and is typically associated with a specific injury involving the head striking or being struck by an object.

Diffuse brain injury is more widespread and is often the result of the skull accelerating or decelerating rapidly. The head does not necessarily make contact with anything.

MTBI can also occur due to a lack of oxygen under a variety of circumstances involving cerebral anoxia or hypoxia.

Cerebral Anoxia and Cerebral Hypoxia

Anoxia and hypoxia are both terms that refer to the lack of oxygen to the brain. Many times the words are used interchangeably. More accurately, the terms delineate degrees of deprivation. Anoxia refers to damage caused by a total lack of oxygen to the brain, while hypoxia describes a decreased or limited amount of oxygen to the brain.

Causes of Anoxic or Hypoxic Brain Trauma

Anoxic brain injury as well as hypoxic brain injury can be caused by brain trauma as a result of carbon monoxide poisoning, drowning, choking, suffocation, head trauma, severe bleeding, drop in blood pressure or stroke.

Anaesthesia errors and other surgical mistakes are also frequently causes of diminished blood supply to the brain, resulting in anoxic brain damage. Brain damage as a result of lack of oxygen is also seen in new-borns, frequently as a result of medical negligence or complications in the delivery of the baby.

Signs and Symptoms of Cerebral Anoxia or Hypoxia

The symptoms of brain damage caused by oxygen deprivation depend on the degree and the length of time that the brain has been deprived of oxygen.

Frequently, individuals will be inattentive, will suffer from poor judgment, and will have memory loss and poor motor coordination.

If the lack of oxygen to the brain lasts for several minutes, an individual's brain cells will begin to die, resulting in permanent brain damage, coma, seizures or even death.

Treatment for Anoxia and Hypoxia

The treatment for anoxia and hypoxia involves restoring an individual's blood pressure and the supply of oxygen to the brain. It may also include blood transfusions, administration of oxygen and medication to control seizure activity.

Brain Damage Following Cerebral Anoxia or Hypoxia

The extent of brain damage depends on the how long the brain was deprived of oxygen. It is well known that it only takes a few minutes of oxygen deprivation for brain cells to begin to die.

The longer the brain has been starved from receiving necessary oxygen, the greater the degree of injury to the brain, or the higher the chance of coma or death. Persons who recover from oxygen loss frequently have memory loss, personality changes, behavioural changes, amnesia, hallucinations and muscle damage.

Unfortunately, where there has been significant oxygen loss, the brain is severely compromised resulting in coma. Since the brain damage is extremely severe, the prospect of a good recovery is very limited.

The Mechanics of a MTBI

The brain is much less solid than most people realise. The consistency is more like gelatine, with the entire structure suspended in cerebrol-spinal fluid. Although the bony skull protects the brain, it can also be part of the mechanism that harms it.

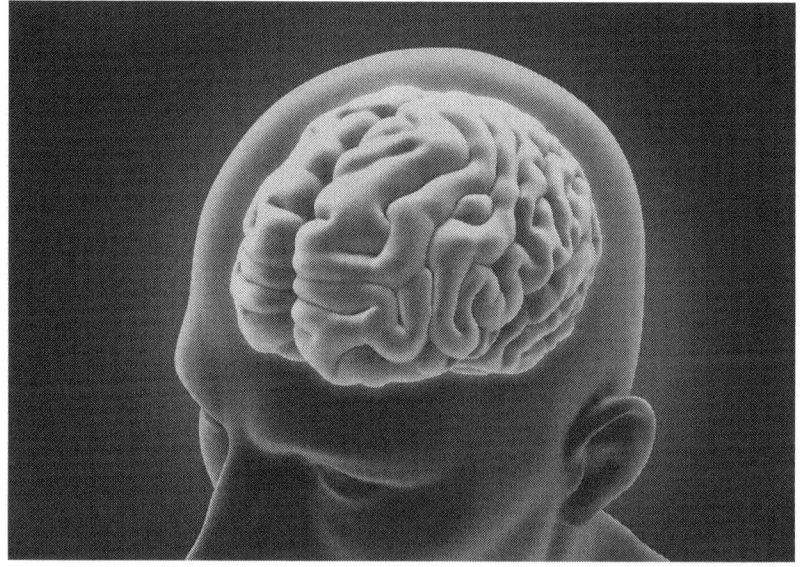

If the head is subject to a sudden and violent blow or movement, either accelerating or decelerating, the brain impacts the rough, uneven interior of the skull.

Both the motion and the impact can cause the nerve cells or axons, which resemble threads, to strain and stretch.

By the same token, when the neck suffers severe and sudden rotation, the twisting motion causes a similar effect. In either case, the placement of the neurons is altered, and the neural cells can even tear.

Both motions — impact and rotation — are forms of concussion.

The disrupted balance of the axons, coupled with swelling, severely interrupts the brain's neurological circuits resulting in significant cognitive issues and physiological damage.

Even more insidious, however, is the effect on the cells' ability to produce the necessary structural proteins to maintain their diameter.

This degradation of axon integrity is thought to explain the delayed symptoms seen consistently in MTBI cases.

During recovery, the cells work to re-establish their balance, but this may require adjusting the original alignments, or creating new ones to compensate.

If this process happens repeatedly, as in the case of serial concussions, the restructuring takes longer each time and each version is less effective than the proceeding one. Twenty percent of people who suffer even a single concussion never fully recover.

Chapter 2 - Brain Injury Measurement

Typically after a head injury some form of neuroimaging is used in an effort to assess the resulting damage. However neither CT scans nor MRI scans will show the kind of damage present in an MTBI, because the effect is to the brain's "white matter" or neuron connections.

Advances in Imaging Technology

New imaging technologies have shown promise in the area of MTBI diagnosis, but the tests are expensive and not widely available.

These technologies include:

- Positron Emission Tomography (PET)

- Single Photon Emission Computerized Tomography (SPECT)

- Functional Magnetic Resonance Imaging (fMRI)

- Diffuse Tensor Imaging (DTI)

Note that your healthcare insurance may not cover tests that are still considered "non-standard."

Neuropsychological Assessment Remains the Standard

In the vast majority of cases, MTBI is identified by assessing the symptoms reported by the patient. This involves tests to measure key areas of brain function including, but not limited to:

- attention span
- memory
- concentration
- language
- mathematical reasoning
- spatial perception
- abstract and organization thinking
- problem solving
- social judgment
- motor abilities
- sensory awareness
- general psychological adjustment

A neuropsychological evaluation is generally the starting point for a program of rehabilitation. It helps medical professionals determine the cognitive areas that have suffered damage, as well as those that are functioning properly.

Scales and Measurement of Functioning

As a means of determining both the extent of a brain injury and the progress of the person's recovery, a variety of measurement scales are employed.

Disability Rating Scale (DRS)

This measurement was developed with both juveniles and adults suffering from moderate to traumatic levels of brain injury. The scale was arrived at in an inpatient rehabilitation setting as an effort to track patients from "coma to community."

The scale runs from 0 to 29, with 0 being no functional impairment, and 29 being a vegetative state. In order for the test to be deemed "reliable," the score must be arrived at while the patient is not anesthetized, recovering from surgical anaesthesia, under the influence of mind-altering drugs, or in the aftermath of a seizure.

The combined findings are intended to provide a global depiction of cognitive and physical impairment or disability.

Functional Independent Measure (FIM)

This scale is a rating of an individual's ability to function independently while performing day-to-day living activities including self-care, the management of elimination needs, movement (including transfers), communication, and social interactions.

The scale runs from 1 to 7, with 1 reflecting total dependence, and 7 complete independence.

Functional Assessment Measure (FAM)

This test was developed as an augmentation of the Functional Independent Measure to specifically address cognitive, behavioural, communication, and community functioning assessment.

The FAM consists of 12 items, which, when added to the 18 items on the FIM form a 30-point scale.

(Note that a slightly different version of FAM is used in the United Kingdom that is regarded as more objective by British clinicians.)

Glasgow Coma Scale

This rating scale is meant as a measurement of initial severity of brain injury generally under emergency room conditions. Patients are assessed for motor, verbal, and eye responses.

A score of 3 indicates severe neurological impairment, with 15 being normal to "near" normal.

Rancho Los Amigos (Original)

This scale is used by rehabilitation teams to assess patterns and stages of recovery from brain injury by level of cognitive functioning. The levels are characterized as:

Level 1 - No Response

Sounds, sights, touch or movement elicits no reaction from the patient. Total assistance is required.

Level 2 - Generalized Response

Sounds, sights, touch or movement elicits slow, inconsistent, and often delayed responses that may include chewing, sweating, rapid breathing, moaning, movement, or changes in blood pressure. Total assistance is required.

Level 3 - Localized Response

The patient is awake at intervals through the day and may move or react specifically to stimuli, although slowly and inconsistently.

Some recognition of family and friends will be present, and there will be an ability to follow simple directions and to respond inconsistently and non-verbally to "yes" and "no" questions. Total assistance is required.

Level 4 - Confused and Agitated

The patient will be both confused and frightened with no understanding of what is happening. Unless restrained, overreactions to stimuli may cause self-harm.

There will be an intense level of focus on basic needs, an inability to concentrate or to follow directions, and intermittent recognition of family and friend. Maximal assistance is required.

Level 5 - Confused and Inappropriate

The patient will be able to pay attention for brief periods, but will be confused and have difficulty making sense of his surroundings. They will not know the date, or understand where they are, nor will they be able to complete simple daily activities without precise instructions.

Long-term memory will be better than short-term, and sensory overload will be a problem. Filling in gaps by making things up (confabulation) is to be expected. Maximal assistance is required.

Level 6 - Confused and Appropriate

Memory and cognitive problems will be present, although the patient will be able to remember the main points of conversations, if not precise details.

There will be an ability to follow a routine with assistance and there will be an awareness of the month and year if not the specific date.

Attention span will be approximately 30 minutes in the absence of distracting stimuli. Self-care is manageable, and there will be awareness that an injury has occurred but this will be more in terms of physical impairment than cognitive.

There is a strong tendency to associate problems with being in the hospital, and a firm conviction that all will be well as soon as they gets home. Moderate assistance is required.

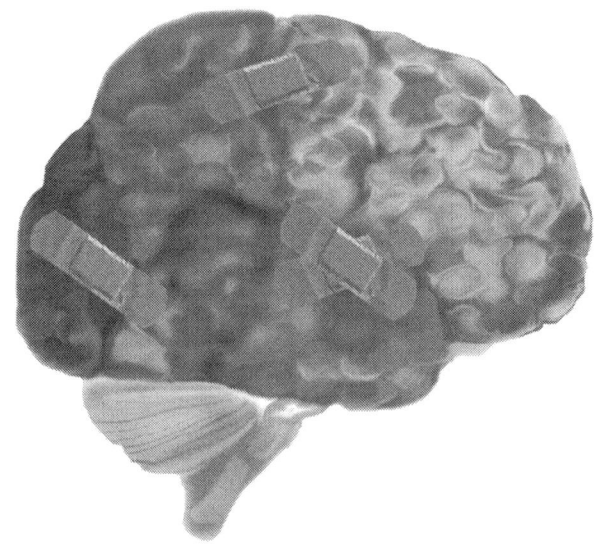

Level 7 - Automatic and Appropriate

These patients can follow a set schedule and maintain routine self-care without help. They will have difficulty making plans, beginning, and completing activities.

Concentration will suffer during distracting or stressful situations, and there may be no realistic understanding that issues with cognition and memory may prevent a return to previous work or living circumstances. Minimal assistance for daily living skills is required.

Level 8 - Purposeful and Appropriate

These patients do understand that they have issues with thinking and memory, they will actively develop compensatory strategies. They will be more flexible and more willing to be evaluated, although their learning will be at a slower rate, which may lead to sensory overload when confronted with difficulties.

Poor judgment in new circumstances can be an issue, and guidance in making decisions is beneficial. The level of cognitive disruption with which these patients deal may not be noticeable to people who did not know them prior to their injury. Stand-by assistance is most appropriate in these cases.

Rancho Los Amigos (Revised)

The revised version of this scale includes the original 8 levels and adds two more:

Level 9 - Purposeful, Appropriate: Stand-By Assistance on Request

These patients shift independently between tasks and can maintain attention and accuracy for two hours at a time. Memory devices to assist with scheduling as well as task lists are helpful, but the person can initiate and carry out all the steps to complete work and household-related projects.

The patient is aware of and acknowledges their disabilities and impairments. They consider the consequences of their decisions and accurately estimate their abilities.

They may grapple with both irritability and depression, and will have a low tolerance level for frustration, but they are able to self-monitor for appropriateness.

Level 10 - Purposeful, Appropriate: Modified Independent

These patients handle multiple tasks well, but will need periodic breaks. They independently procure memory assistance devices, and independently initiate home and work projects. They anticipate problems related to their impairments and compensate accordingly.

They retain the ability to recognize and address the needs and feeling of others, responding in an appropriate manner. Periodic depression and irritability will be present, with low frustration levels. Their behaviour in social situations is both consistent and appropriate.

A Caution Regarding Cognitive Testing

With all cognitive testing, it is important to realise that results can vary widely per individual. The variability of measurement can be due to the environment in which the test is administered, or be a consequence of something that is simply "stuck" in the person's memory.

As an example, many people who suffer with Alzheimer's disease are capable of achieving perfect cognitive scores in the early stages of the disease even when their behavioural symptoms are obvious.

The explanation is that they have simply retained, for whatever reason, the necessary information to answer the test questions.

All cognitive test results, regardless of the degree of brain injury, must be viewed with some amount of caution, and balanced carefully against actual functioning abilities.

Emerging Awareness of MTBI

In part, due to the wars in Iraq and Afghanistan, brain trauma has come to the forefront of the public consciousness. Severe brain injuries are the "signature" wound of these conflicts, a fact which has led to significant improvements in treatment methods and long-term prognosis for successful recovery.

An awareness of the effects of MTBI, however, especially the cumulative consequences of multiple injuries like concussions, has been slower to develop both in medical circles and in the general population.

These consequences can involve complex emotional and psychological reactions to a traumatic incident, including post-traumatic stress disorder. Sorting out the effects of the injury and the long-term emotional effects of the trauma of the injury, make an accurate diagnosis even more difficult.

Since 2000, there have been 220,430 cases of TBI (Traumatic Brain Injury) among U.S. servicemen. Of those, 60% to 80% were actually MTBIs, a fact that really did not fully come to light until 2007, and was not passed on to line commanders until 2009. At that time, officers were apprised of the fact that MTBI could result in:

- diminished marksmanship
- slowed reaction times
- decreased concentration

In light of those findings, the criteria for sending soldiers back into a combat setting had to be reconsidered and revised.

Kathy Helmick, Deputy Director of the Defence Centres of Excellence, speaking at the 4th Annual Trauma Spectrum Conference in December 2011 was quoted in an article for U.S. Medicine, saying *"Mild TBI remains little understood and hard to diagnose."*

"There's a dire necessity to find an objective marker for concussion," Helmick said. *"We have been very much challenged and prompted by Congress to find this objective marker beyond the clinical judgment."*

Promising avenues for better diagnosis include measurements of:

- papillary response and visual tracking
- serum, saliva, and skin biomarkers
- diffuse tensor imaging
- electrophysiological parameters

Currently, however, doctors are still, for the most part, just talking to their patients and trying to make a diagnostic determination based on what they hear.

One of the greatest hurdles to diagnosing MTBI is the patients themselves. Many hide their problems and find ways to compensate for the cognitive deficits they are fighting, or the patient simply does not know what is wrong with them.

Since many of the symptoms of MTBI are delayed, and the effects of cumulative MTBI are poorly understood, unknown numbers of people face this condition alone and isolated.

Case Study: Falling - The Most Common Cause of MTBI

On June 16 2011, Heather Marsh, DCoE Strategic Communications wrote an article for the Defence Centres of Excellence for Psychological Health and Traumatic Brain Injury (DCoE), entitled "My Discovery of Mild Traumatic Brain Injury," in which she describes her own "cluelessness" of the topic.

In March 2011, Marsh fell, face forward on a hardwood floor, an incident that required a trip to the emergency room, and five stitches. She went home and thought her bruised ego was really the worst part of the whole thing.

Then, over a period of about ten days, she experienced frightening feelings of helplessness and disorientation. Marsh spoke with her DCoE colleagues, including one who was a former chief of neurology, and realised she had suffered a concussion.

In spite of where she worked and with whom, Marsh had no idea that falls are the leading cause of mild traumatic brain injury (MTBI).

Marsh experienced a wide range of symptoms, including a sense of anxious fear from simply watching sunlight flickering through the trees on a drive home. *"I felt a sudden rush of panic as if I was intoxicated,"* she wrote. *"I felt disoriented and blinded all at once."*

Thankfully she was able to pull over to the side of the road and collect herself to finish the drive home. The incident left her wondering, however, how returning American veterans must cope with intense sensory overload in the face of multiple MTBIs sustained in combat.

Marsh's concussion symptoms resolved naturally over time, but she came away from her brush with MTBI realizing that not everyone knows how to explain when something is just "wrong."

Marsh benefitted from working with experts who helped her to understand what was happening to her body; otherwise, she might well have remained silent and afraid, with no concrete information about her injury.

Source: Marsh, Heather. "My Discovery of Mild Traumatic Brain Injury," 16 June 11, Defence Centres for Excellence, http://www.dcoe.health.mil/blog/11-06-16/My_Discovery_of_Mild_Traumatic_Brain_Injury.aspx (Accessed June 2013).

Chapter 3 - Diagnosing Minimal and Moderate Brain Trauma

Unlike other medical conditions, there is no perfect biomarker to diagnose a traumatic brain injury at any level. A biomarker is defined as a specific physical trait used to measure or indicate the effects or progress of a disease or condition.

To be classed as "perfect," a biomarker for TBI would have to meet five highly specific criteria:

- Indicate the pathology of the damage to the brain.

- Appear in some biological fluid, most likely blood, within hours of the injury causing the TBI.

- Exhibit a correlation with measurements obtained from neuroimages and neurological scoring.

- Predict the outcome of the course of the TBI.

- Allow for follow-up monitoring and adjustment of therapies and medications.

The absence of a "perfect" biomarker, however, does not mean that researchers have not made significant strides in developing quantifiable tests for diagnosing brain trauma.

The Evolution of Blood-Based Diagnostics for TBI

Over the past five years, scientists have attempted to derive a measurement from cellular proteins in the blood, secreted proteins and peptides, and proteolytic fragments (created from the breakdown of proteins.) The first clinical trials resulted in very limited performance and a failure to meet the five major requirements.

In 2011, however, a study published in the Annals of Emergency Medicine, pointed to raised levels of acidic protein in the blood of patients with TBI. The authors suggested that a test for the protein administered within four hours of the initial injury could provide an accurate measure of the level of head trauma present.

The most reliable indicator that has surfaced since that time is the serum protein S100B, which is present normally only in the brain. If it is found in the bloodstream, the blood-brain barrier has been compromised and a brain injury has occurred, even if there are no symptoms evident.

The blood-brain barrier serves as a dynamic, protective interface, separating both the brain and the central nervous system from harmful chemicals traveling in the circulatory system.

Looking at a serum protein in isolation may point to the presence of brain trauma, but the real goal is what the authors of "Blood-Based Diagnostics of Traumatic Brain Injuries" (Expert Review of Molecular Diagnostics, January 2011) called "a multimarker strategy that could be useful in refining risk stratification and for categorizing patients with TBI."

More pointedly, however, the same study concluded with this sobering assessment:

"The seriousness and complexity of the problems posed by TBI have been underestimated. Current classification systems are no longer sufficient. No clinical method is available for an accurate assessment of the severity of injury and outcome in patients with TBI, especially in mild TBI, since mild TBI patients have only subtle disturbances."

Brain Injury Testing in Professional Sports

Researchers at the Cleveland Clinic and at the University of Rochester are actively studying long-term brain changes in professional football players.

These athletes, according to work published by the National Institute for Occupational Safety and Health in Cincinnati in Neurology (September 2012), face an elevated risk for the development of neurodegenerative disease including, but not limited to, Parkinson's and Alzheimer's.

Dr. Damir Janigro, the director of cerebrovascular research at the Cleveland Clinic's Lerner Research Institute was quoted by Medical News Today in March 2013, *"Much attention is being paid to concussions among football players and the big hits that cause them, but research shows that more common 'sub-concussive' hits appear to cause damage, too."*

In 67 football players involved in the Cleveland Clinic study, S100B levels increased, even though none of the players were diagnosed with a concussion. Four of the participants tested positive for a brain disorder in their measurable autoimmune responses according to the blood work performed.

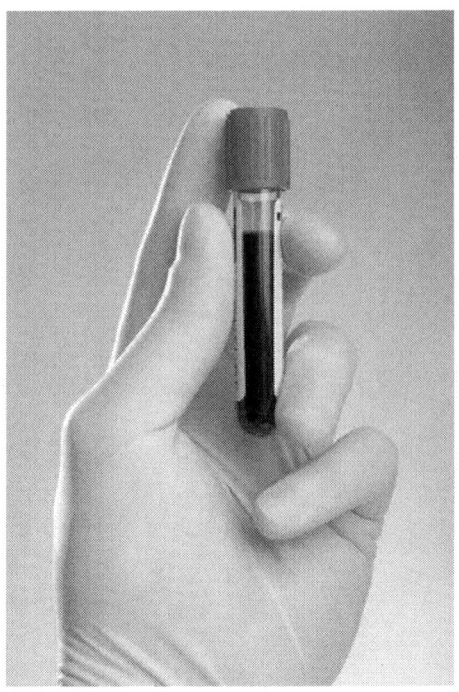

When S100B is present in the blood, the body creates an autoimmune response. Antibodies are released, and find their way to the brain where they negatively affect the tissues causing long-term brain damage.

In addition to undergoing blood tests for S100B levels, the players received brain scans, and were tested for motor control, reaction time, balance, and memory.

Approximately 40% of all professional football players in the United States suffer at least one concussion a year. The S100B test has proven to be a good indicator of this level of brain trauma, and at a cost of just $40 / £27 compared to much more expensive and less predictive techniques like CT scans or MRI scans.

Blood Testing for Concussion Used in Europe, not U.S.

Unfortunately, blood tests for S100B, though widely used in Europe as an emergency room screening protocol for concussion, have not been equally accepted in the United States.

This disappointing fact comes even in the face of high demand for better assessment tools for MTBI, especially among the parents of youth athletes.

This growing concern stems primarily from the now well-established scientific link between long-term degenerative brain diseases and concussion, highlighted by the tragic suicides of NFL athletes like former San Diego Charger linebacker Junior Seau who shot himself in 2012. His autopsy indicated the presence of chronic traumatic encephalopathy, or CTE, caused by repeated blows to the head during his years as a professional player.

In an article by Bill Pennington, "A New Way to Care for Young Brains" that appeared in The New York Times on May 5, 2013, Dr. William Meehan, co-founder of the Sports Concussion Clinic at Boston's Children's Hospital, said, "It used to be a completely different scene, with a child's father walking in reluctantly to tell us, 'He's fine; this concussion stuff is nonsense.' It's totally the opposite now. A kid has one concussion, and the parents are very worried about how he'll function at 50 years old."

CTE, which causes a cascade of symptoms similar to Alzheimer's, including marked changes in behaviour, major depression, memory loss, and issues with impulse control.

Currently, CTE can only be conclusively diagnosed post-mortem, but it has been found in both professional athletes and young athletes who have committed suicide.

The problem has commanded enough public attention in the United States that 47 states and the District of Columbia have now passed the Lystedt Law. This law requires school-age athletes who have sustained a concussion to have written authorization from a doctor (often one trained in concussion management) before they can be cleared to play again.

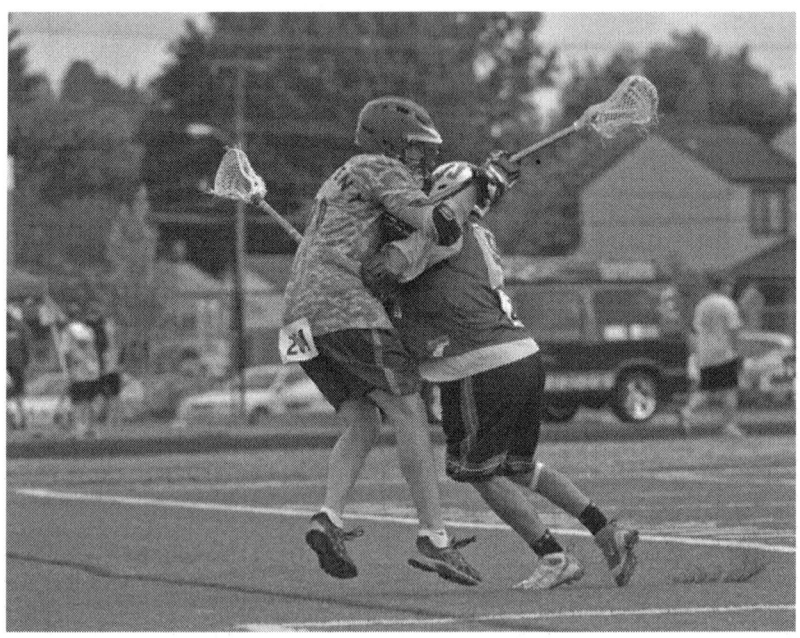

A more difficult aspect of the problem lies with the athletes themselves, however. In a study conducted by researchers at Cincinnati Children's school, just under half of high school athletes surveyed said they would not report symptoms of concussion to their coach in order to get back into the game. The majority of those same players admitted that they were aware of the risk of serious injury from such a decision.

Emerging Picture of the Seriousness of MTBI

The research into a blood-based testing protocol for MTBI has proven that repeated traumas to the head, even in the absence of diagnosed concussion, weaken the blood brain barrier. If that barrier is compromised, damage to the brain of some degree appears inevitable.

The complete ramifications of such injuries may not be apparent, however, for decades as shown by newly gained insights into CTE. Even in cases of "complete recovery" from a concussion, the brain will never be the same.

Responses to this problem have ranged from efforts to develop better protective head gear, to the rising prevalence of "youth concussion clinics" adjacent to major hospitals in the United States.

The most recent studies suggest, however, that even heavier, high-tech helmets do not mitigate the risk of concussion. In a study released in July 2013 that looked at 1,300 high school football players at 36 different schools, players wearing traditional helmets enjoyed the same level of protection against concussion as those equipped with newer models.

The author of the study, Dr. Timothy McGuine, research coordinator the University of Wisconsin Health Sports Medicine Centre in Madison said, "The helmet technology is advanced as it can be. They've done a wonderful job. We don't have skull fractures in football. But I don't know how much padding can be put in to prevent the brain from sloshing around inside the cranium."

(**Source**: "Concussion Prevention: Pass on Pricey Football Helmets, Study Suggests," MedlinePlus, 15 July 2013,

Only in Europe, however, have doctors embraced blood testing as a truly predictive way to identify elevated protein levels as an indicator of "mild" brain injury.

Until such tests are universally accepted and used to prevent re-injury, the more than 1.5 million concussions that occur in the U.S. each year, and those that happen as a result of contact sports around the world will continue unabated.

The task of recovering from MTBI and living with its consequences are the price patients must pay while medical science plays catch-up to fully understand and to address a condition so erroneously characterized as "mild."

Case Study: Youngest Case of Chronic Traumatic Encephalopathy on Record

In 2009, clinical researchers at the Centre for the Study of Traumatic Encephalopathy at the Boston University School of Medicine disclosed their finding of the degenerative brain condition in the autopsy results of an 18 year old multi-sport athlete.

This individual, whose name was withheld at the request of his parents, is the youngest person ever to be diagnosed with the degenerative brain disorder.

Had the boy lived, he would have developed early onset dementia, like that presenting in numerous NFL athletes like former San Diego Charger's linebacker Junior Seau who likely suffered a staggering 1,500 concussions in his 15-year professional football career.

Dr. Ann McKee, a neurologist and head of the brain bank at BU said that of thousands of post-mortem exams she has conducted, traumatic encephalopathy has only been present in athletes, not in the general population.

The 18-year-old suffered numerous concussions playing high school football and other contact sports, and had played contact sports in the week before his death. The details of his death were not disclosed save to say the circumstances did not involve head trauma or violence.

Former Harvard football player and professional wrestler Chris Nowinski, co-director of the BU centre and author of Head Games: Football's Concussion Crisis said, "This should be a wakeup call, especially to parents, coaches and league administrators. We're exposing more than 1 million kids to early-onset brain damage and we don't know yet how to prevent it."

Sources: Bob Hohler, "Major Breakthrough in Concussion Crisis: Researchers Find Signs of Degenerative Brain Disease in an 18-Year-Old High School Player," The Boston Globe, 27 January 2009, http://www.boston.com/sports/other_sports/articles/2009/01/27/major_breakthrough_in_concussion_crisis/?page=full (Accessed July 2013); "Case Study: 18 Year Old High School Football Player," BU Centre for the Study of Traumatic Encephalopathy, http://www.bu.edu/cste/case-studies/18-year-old/ (Accessed July 2013).

Chapter 4 – The Journey Towards Recovery

There is no set pattern of recovery from brain injury. Each case of MTBI is as individual as the person experiencing the injury. Sometimes the neurons in the brain heal. Sometimes they don't. Regardless, recovery from MTBI is a slow process.

Often you will face the incomprehension and even insensitivity of the people around you, who think you look just fine. You will always face your own frustration because you, more than anyone else, will be aware of the fact that you are far from "fine."

There are general guidelines and insights about MTBI to help you, your family, and your friends, but the journey will be uniquely your own.

Your Injury May Initially Be Dismissed Out of Hand

Let's say that you're in an automobile accident. Perhaps your vehicle is struck from behind and you're first thrown forward in the car before your head snaps backward.

This motion is called coup and coutrecoup. First, your brain makes impact when it shoots forward and hits the front of your skull. Then, it is injured again when it snaps backward and strikes the rear of the skull.

The car comes to a stop. You're still conscious and you're not bleeding, but already have a headache. In general, however, you're just relieved to be alive.

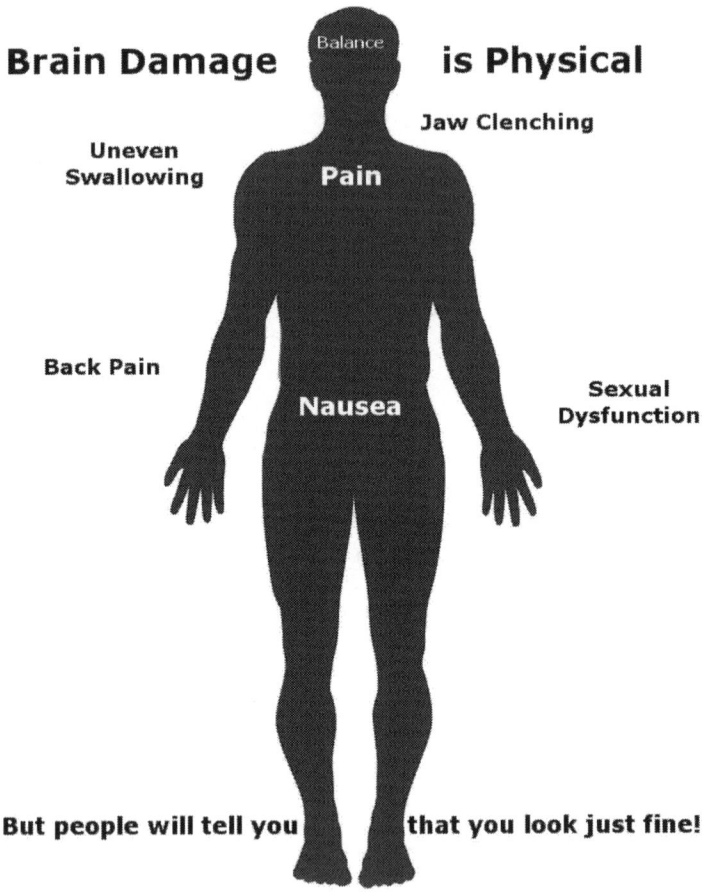

Brain Damage Balance **is Physical**

Jaw Clenching

Uneven
Swallowing

Pain

Back Pain

Sexual
Dysfunction

Nausea

But people will tell you that you look just fine!

Next, the Paramedics arrive. You know your name. You know how many fingers the tech is holding up. Just to be safe, however, you agree to go to the emergency room.

There, you receive a CT scan or maybe an MRI scan. There's no bleeding. You're feeling a little "banged up," but you're coherent. The doctor gives you two aspirin and sends you home. He may or may not tell you that you have a concussion.

If he does diagnose concussion, his advice will likely be that you should do as little as possible for 2 or 3 weeks until your brain has a chance to heal.

During that time, you should limit all visual and auditory stimuli as much as possible. Essentially, do nothing.

The next morning you wake up feeling like you've come down with the worst case of flu imaginable. Over the next week, your symptoms just get worse. You want to sleep a lot. You're depressed, grieving even, and you can't tell people what happened in the accident.

You get confused when you try, and break down. Your wife and friends are kind. They assume you're just upset, frustrated. It will pass. But then it doesn't. There's a ringing in your ears. It hurts to think. You can't sleep. Maybe you stutter or search for words.

Light hurts your eyes, sound, your ears, so you find some place cool and quiet and isolate yourself. Reading a book to pass the time doesn't work because two minutes after you've read a page you don't remember what it says.

Food smells awful to you. Colours are too bright. Every noise grates on your nerves. Two weeks go by and then comes the day when you think you're better, so you try to rouse yourself to get something done.

You decide you'll go to the store down the street. An hour after you pull out of your driveway, you're wandering in circles, crying, lost, with no idea where you are.

It takes you a week to get over that incident, and then you quietly buy a GPS. You use it to find your way around your own town daily, because you get confused so easily — not just about directions, but about everything. Simple questions throw you into a panic, especially if there's any pressure to answer quickly.

Ashamed and afraid about what's happening to you, you try to hide your symptoms, but the cognitive strain becomes too severe.

Finally, you just short circuit. With too much information flooding your system and no ability to filter and make sense of it all, you have to admit that something is very, very wrong.

As insane as it may sound for anyone to have to go through that level of physical and emotional pain to have their injury recognized as valid, some variation on this scenario happens to MTBI sufferers every day.

Even when you reach a level of being completely unable to function, don't necessarily expect medical professionals to behave as you will rightfully expect they should. It is a sad fact of MTBI that more doctors are uninformed than informed about the real severity of the problem.

In the face of potential misunderstanding from the doctors who are supposed to be helping you, it may be only your loved ones and friends who really understand that something is NOT right.

The severity of MTBI has only been truly recognized over the past 5 years, and long-term treatment and management of the condition is still at a shockingly archaic level of development. This lag in proper medical response only makes this condition more maddening.

Brain Injuries Present in Physical Ways

Even in the absence of overt bodily injury in cases of MTBI the effects of the injury will manifest in decidedly physical ways. As if the cognitive and functional fall out were not sufficiently severe, you may also find yourself dealing with:

- Balance issues including dizziness and vertigo
- Nausea and stomach upset
- Neck/shoulder pain, including headaches and scalp pain
- Jaw clenching and grinding (day and night)
- Back pain
- Uneven swallowing and choking on saliva or food

It is not unusual for a person's eyeglass prescription to be different following MTBI or for women to experience a disrupted hormone cycle.

It would be a mistake to think of MTBI as a head injury per se because the brain is in charge of all the body's systems.

When something is wrong in "command central," the effects filter throughout the entire body. These symptoms do regularize over time, but while they are present they only make you feel even "crazier."

Balance Issues

People who have suffered an MTBI may not be able to walk a straight line or to close their eyes and touch the end of their nose. Sudden motions will likely bring on a wave of nausea, or the effect may be completely random and unpredictable. Until balance issues begin to resolve, don't drive or use any kind of machinery.

In general, move slowly and try to avoid sudden shifts in posture, like standing too quickly from a sitting position, or looking up suddenly. Sometimes wearing dark glasses both indoors and out will help, since light flashes may trigger a bout of dizziness.

Vision Problems

Extreme sensitivity to light is one of the most often cited results of MTBI, followed by blurred vision, black spots, or areas of the visual field that seem blurred as if they were smeared with thick grease. Your ability to focus your eyes and to use your peripheral vision may also be affected. Again, dark glasses help and it's best to avoid using machinery.

If these visual problems continue after several weeks, visit your ophthalmologist. It is possible that you may need glasses, or if you already wear glasses that your prescription will have to be altered.

In a few months you may have to go through another examination as your eyes normalize, but since the effects of visual disruptions are so acute, better to pay the price of an extra pair of glasses than try to live in a world you can't see.

Hormones in Disarray

Women who experience an MTBI will likely see a disruption of their menstrual cycle, which may change in frequency, flow, or duration. Hormones, however, affect all the body's systems from sleep to digestion.

Hormonal fallout can also be seen in the immune system, which may be less capable of fending off infectious agents. People with MTBI can easily develop colds and coughs that hang on for months, and women are highly susceptible to yeast infections.

Sexual Dysfunction

Sexual response is one of the most complicated of all bodily reactions. Multiple systems have to co-operate for an individual to be interested in intimacy. It is quite common for a person with MTBI to lose their sex drive or not to be able to function sexually. Basically, the brain just doesn't have enough energy to manage all the complicated processes involved.

Do not try to rush this part of your recovery. Sexual interest and function may return slowly, although this area of your life, like many others, may be different after MTBI. Both you and your partner will need to be patient with one another. If possible, don't let issues of self-esteem make the problem even more frustrating. Return to intimacy in stages.

It is important for partners to understand that hypersensitivity may extend to physical touch no matter how loving. What once felt good may now be unpleasant.

Partners need to listen and talk, allowing new paths of intimacy to develop. It may be necessary for individuals to experiment on their own to discover what now works and then to share that information with their partner.

Since sex is an aerobic activity and stamina is low after MTBI, try not to be frightened by rapid heart rate or shortness of breath. Just slow down, do not, however, seek the aid of alcoholic beverages to "take the edge off." Alcohol inhibits sexual function in perfectly healthy people, but can make the situation far, far worse for someone with MTBI.

The flip side of disinterest or dysfunction in the bedroom is inappropriate behaviour or disinhibition. You not only want it, you want it all the time, and not necessarily at appropriate times. This issue is generally hardest on your partner.

If sexually inappropriate behaviour is a problem, seek the help of a professional counsellor. Again, this is a temporary effect, but one with an enormous potential for embarrassment and damaged relations if not handled.

Getting the Help of Trauma Specialists is Imperative

More and more people suffering with MTBI are turning to the aid of neurotrauma case managers, speech and language therapists, life coaches, and other trauma professionals. These people, working on the cutting edge of MTBI recovery strategies and understand that you don't just sleep off a brain injury.

These therapy specialists help MTBI patients create the optimum environment for recovery by identifying and implementing coping strategies. These could include, but are certainly not limited to:

- Recognizing the difference between sticking with a task, and needing to stop. The brain isn't a muscle that can be strengthened by working harder. Overdoing can actually hinder the progress of recovery from MTBI.

- Carrying a notebook to keep track of the thousands of little bits of information we all need in our day-to-day lives. Something as simple as having your own personal reference book can cut down on the frustration that will often trigger a crisis episode in an MTBI patient's day.

- Scheduling every day common tasks with adequate time to complete things at your new pace. Leaving things to the last minute will only increase stress and anxiety. Planning in advance and staggering tasks will make life more manageable and help you to feel more in control.

- Learning to rehearse stressful situations. Therapists provide MTBI patients with a place to practice how they will respond to situations they find distressing, like simply being asked, "How are you?" Because social filters often erode with brain injury, the patient may struggle with how much information to share and an inability to formulate a socially acceptable innocuous answer like, "I'm doing better."

- Finding new stress relieving activities. Many people with MTBI find that the endorphins released during exercise are incredibly helpful in managing their levels of stress. Others like activities that give them a sense of restoring order, like putting together jigsaw puzzles or doing something creative.

Trauma specialists also work with friends and family to help them understand the hugely important role they play in the life of a person recovering from MTBI. Significant others need to learn how to anticipate likely reactions and make mitigating responses.

People with MTBI grapple with a great deal of guilt about not doing "enough," like returning to work, while being overwhelmed with a sense that everything is too much. It is important for them to know they are not alone as a tendency toward self-isolation is very strong in these cases.

Family and friends will have their own share of frustrations. The person they know and love is not acting and reacting in the ways to which they are accustomed, and they too will be scared, anxious, and even angry.

Exploring the Fallout of MTBI

Although it cannot be stressed strongly enough that every case of MTBI is unique to the individual, and must be treated uniquely, there are common denominators that surface in varying combinations with this type of injury.

Disruptions in Normal Thought Patterns

Most of us have no reason to ever dissect the way we think, or to separate the multiple components involved in taking in and processing information.

This may mean anything from understanding the language that is being spoken, to working out a simple math problem at lunch, to getting the amount of tip right.

People with MTBI, however, grapple with difficulties in very specific cognitive areas that affect every facet of their daily lives including (but not limited to):

- attention
- concentration
- memory
- reasoning
- planning
- understanding
- speech and language

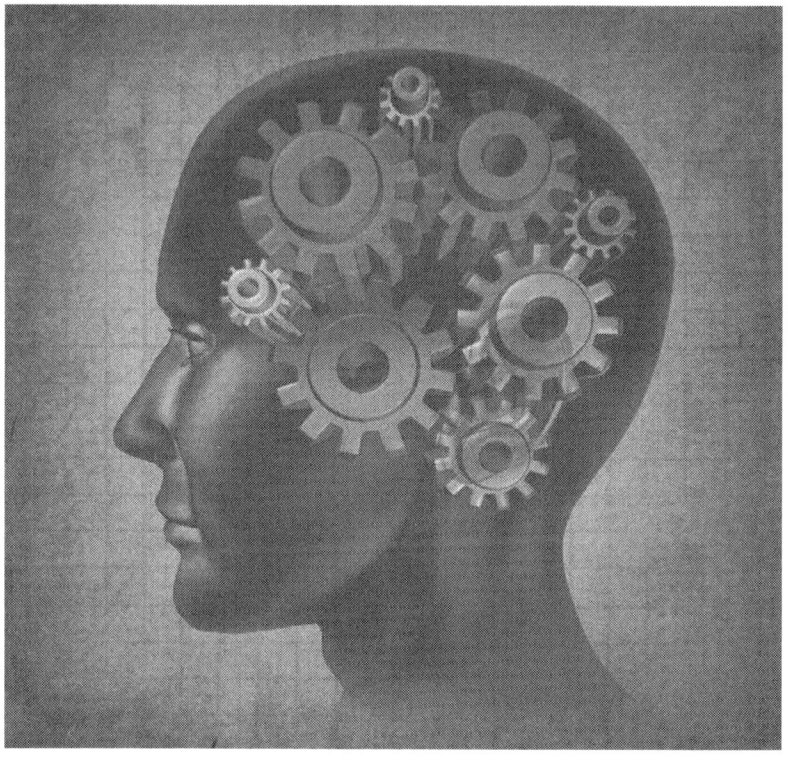

These mechanical problems spill out into a range of functional struggles from anger management to sexual dysfunction.

The Interrelated Nature of Thought

We take for granted the ability to easily shift and redirect our attention and concentration during our every waking moment. The sensory overload MTBI patients face stems directly from the absence of such filters that regulate sensations like sound and touch.

Some people with MTBI say that for the first time in their lives they are actually aware of their feet touching the ground as they walk. Others, who always loved summer nights, suddenly find the sound of chirping crickets unbearably loud and grating.

Two cognitive functions come into play in these situations. First is attention, the ability to selectively focus on specific input the senses are receiving. Normally, we can choose to ignore or tune out one thing in favour of another. We decide where our attention will be directed.

In some instances, however, we also remain alert to the presence of a potential stimulus in the background, for instance the sound of a baby waking up from its nap.

In moments of concentration, we achieve a state of sustained attention for the purpose of acquiring and retaining new information. Studying for an exam is a good example.

For some people with MTBI, they will not be able to listen for the sound of a baby awakening and read a textbook – and if they did manage to do so, the chances are they would not remember much of what they were reading.

We all suffer from inattention from time to time, for instance, instantly forgetting the name of someone to whom we've been introduced at a dinner party. But an MTBI sufferer might ask a waiter, "How much is the check?" and fail to remember the amount long enough to get the money out of their wallet.

Even more disconcerting for some people is the phenomenon known as "Swiss cheese effect," which is seen in long-term memory deficits and is an inability to consistently retrieve previously learned information.

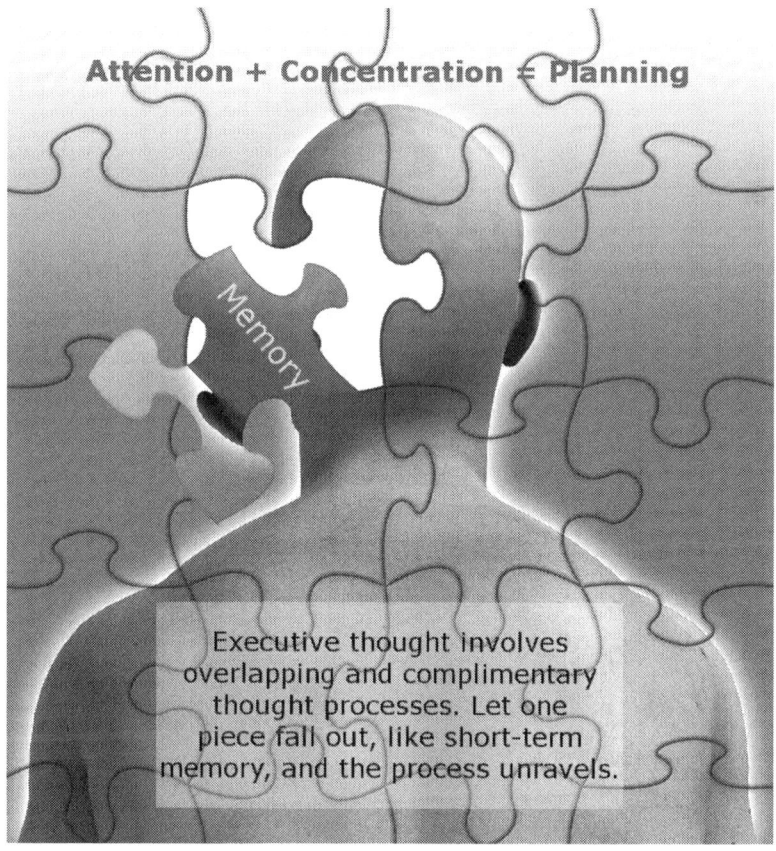

Attention + Concentration = Planning

Memory

Executive thought involves overlapping and complimentary thought processes. Let one piece fall out, like short-term memory, and the process unravels.

A person suffering this kind of cognitive deficit might remember that Abraham Lincoln was president, but not be able to supply a single piece of information about the American Civil War over which Lincoln presided.

With these kinds of short and long-term memory gaps, MTBI patients also find task management difficult because their concept of time has been altered as well as their ability to appropriately allocate their time. They have problems judging how much time is required to complete particular chores, and tracking due dates eludes them.

For these and other reasons, executive functions overwhelm an MTBI sufferer. How do you tell the importance of one thing over another? How do you prioritize? Since doing two things at once throws the person into overload, they often lose their ability to initiate action because they literally do not know where to begin.

In previously decisive and focused individuals, the inability to make a decision is terrifying and excruciating. In their fear, they become defensive and secretive, doing everything possible to hide their struggles from those around them, especially the people with whom they work or live. If the person is also experiencing communication deficits it can easily feel like their world is collapsing.

Chapter 5 - When Words Fail You

Multiple regions of the brain control the processes that allow us not just to speak, but also to interpret the ebb and flow of conversation and to keep up with nuances of meaning. MTBI can cause problems with:

- Articulation
- Fluency
- Attentiveness
- Interpretation

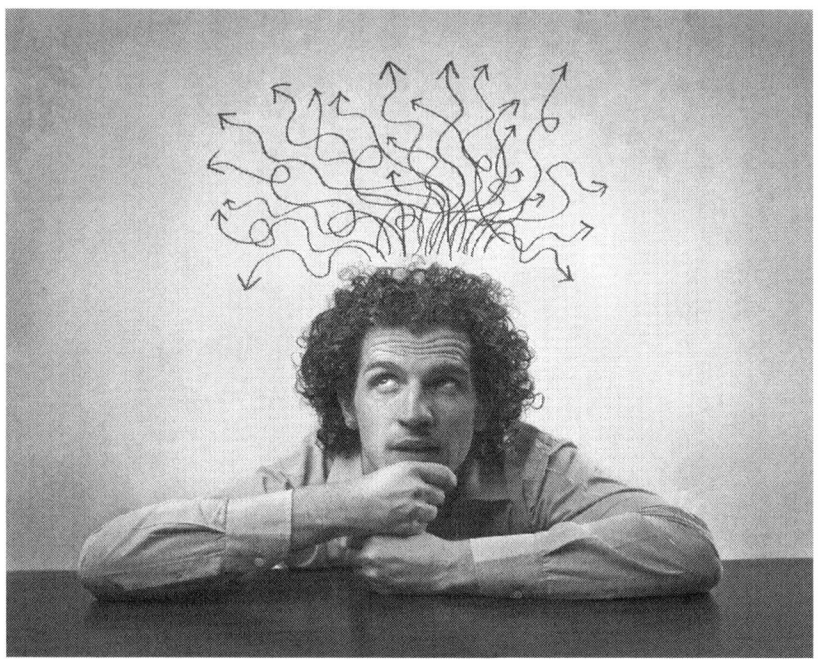

Additionally, if the damage is to the right temporal lobe of the brain, the patient may no longer be able to pick up on and correctly respond to non-verbal communication involving eye contact, expression, posture, and gestures.

Specific speech disruptions typically present are:

- Verbal Apraxia: This condition sounds like stuttering and reflects the speaker's inability to produce words on command.

- Dysarthria: This is the inability to actually move the muscles needed to form and pronounce words.

- Dysfluency: This is the actual technical term for stuttering, a form of speech characterized by hesitant stammering and partially formed words.

- Dysphasia – partial loss in generation of speech and sometimes also in its comprehension.

As a concurrent language problem, aphasia may also be present. This is, generally speaking, an inability to understand and to express words in their correct context. For instance, a patient might need to go to the bathroom but ask to go to the store.

There are three major forms of aphasia with some distinct sub-sets.

- Expressive aphasia involves sentence structure, spelling, verbal reasoning and rate of speech.

  A typical form is Broca's Aphasia. The person can understand what is being said to them, but cannot respond fluently and instead uses single words and gestures to get their meaning across.

  Inappropriate word choice or grammar confusion is called "neologism," and "anomia" is the inability to correctly name familiar objects.

Other variations include dysnomia (groping for words), fluent (talking rapidly with little meaningful content), conductive (halting speech), and perserverative (uncontrolled repetition).

- Receptive aphasia refers to problems with reading and interpreting both written and spoken language.

Articulation may be normal, but when others speak to you, it will be as if you are hearing a foreign language. If you are able to comprehend portions of what is being said, there will be such broad gaps that you are still unable to respond.

Other forms include paraphasia (the use of partial words), and alexia (an inability to read).

- Mixed aphasia merges both problems with language, comprehension and expression.

Coping with Language and Speech Problems

In most cases of MTBI, articulation problems and stuttering resolve on their own in 3 months or less, with language deficits fading or improving over time, generally with the help of a professional speech therapist.

Therapists understand how to help you retrain the speech centres in the brain, and they are able to monitor your progress, adjusting techniques accordingly. This may involve work with a psychologist or psychotherapist to mitigate the very natural and reasonable frustration that accompanies these issues.

Some things you can do to cope more effectively with language and speech deficits include (but are not limited to):

- Making a conscious effort to relax with deep breathing to help cut down on stuttering.

- Conduct important conversations and visits in a stress-free environment with fewer distractions to increase your ability to comprehend what is being said and to respond appropriately.

- Learning to visualize the word you want to use as if it were on a chalkboard in your mind. This will let you pick a synonym that you are able to say.

- Develop prearranged signals with friends and loved ones so you will know when you're going off on a conversational tangent.

- Don't try to hide your problems. That will only increase your discomfort and embarrassment.

- If you have a normal tendency to be outspoken, curb that for now. When people with MTBI get in stressful situations they both lose their temper and lose their ability to express themselves. That's one powerful recipe for frustration!

Get creative with the ways you work on your communication skills. Turn the sound down on the TV and see if you can interpret what characters are doing based on their expressions and other non-verbal cues.

Keep a journal or try drawing to find other ways to express what you are thinking and feeling while your language skills are improving.

As frustrating as this part of your recovery will be, try to remember that this is a temporary phase. If possible, look at your own garbled mistakes with a dash of humour.

Anchorman Bob Woodward, during an interview, recounted the day when he and his wife waited hours for a cable TV repairman from the company Viacom. In his annoyance and frustration, Woodward exclaimed, "When will that Viagra man get here!"

A Broader Pattern of Symptoms

Other symptoms MTBI patients report include:

- Crushing fatigue and loss of energy, especially in the first few weeks after the injury.

- Personality and behavioural changes generally associated with anger management and impulse control.

- Post-traumatic stress disorder characterized by re-living the events of the injury or experiencing negative responses to similar circumstances.

- Amnesia, sometimes about the event, or about the period of time immediately before and after the event.

- Anxiety and panic attacks that may lead to agoraphobia, the fear of leaving home.

- Depression, mood swings, and anger that make social interaction difficult.

- Sexual dysfunction that may be physical and/or emotional in nature.

- Obsessive-compulsive tendencies in an attempt to "manage" your condition.

Sometimes people with MTBI actually develop mood swings severe enough to be characterized as manic-depressive.

A Word About Fatigue

It is crucial to understand the physical nature of fatigue as it relates to energy, which is made up of the physical, emotional, and cognitive elements as well as our "reserves." Listen to your inner voice!

When you're getting tired, stop and take a break. This is nothing to be ashamed of. Fatigue may well continue for the rest of your life after MTBI.

Everyone Wants the Impossible, an Exact Prognosis

Due to the completely individual character of each case of MTBI, offering blanket estimates of an exact prognosis is neither possible nor fair. To suggest that any patient will be at X point after X number of weeks is not a real-world scenario in these cases.

Traditionally medical science has suggested that people who suffer a concussion recover in a matter of weeks. This may be true in that any lingering effects of the concussion are sufficiently minor as to be negligible in their impact on the person's lifestyle.

The mitigating factor in many cases of concussion is the presence or absence of re-injury. In instances of serial concussions, each injury makes it less possible for the brain to repair itself and deficits become progressively glaring.

In severe or multiple cases of MTBI, some patients may work for years and never reach a full level of functional return.

In all cases of brain injury, it is generally accepted that the long-term window of opportunity for recovery is 2-3 years. If a function can be regained, it will be regained in that period.

Increasingly, research indicates that the prognosis of recovery for MTBI is dependent on numerous factors, including age.

A study released in July 2013 by researchers at the University of Oregon and the University of British Columbia showed continued disruption of executive functions in teenagers with concussion 2 months after the initial injury.

This is nearly twice as long as the duration reported in young adults. In this population, cognitive functioning begins to improve in two weeks to one month.

A similar study conducted in 2012 found ongoing neuropsychological deficits in concussed adolescents at least 6 months after the injury.

The authors speculated a greater vulnerability to concussion among adolescents due to the rapid growth of the frontal region of the brain during this phase of life.

(**Source**: Lindsay Barton, "Effects of Concussion on Higher Cognitive Function Persist In Teens, Study Says," Moms Team, 5 June 2013, http://www.momsteam.com/health-safety/effects-concussion-higher-cognitive-function-persist-in-teens-study-says , accessed July 2013.)

In truth, it is much easier to assign milestones to traumatic brain injury than to cases of MTBI because the latter are so much more highly individualized and more difficult to predict.

At some point, patients who have been working for months and seeing little progress may have to face the prospect of what a limited recovery will mean for them.

They may only be able to resume their careers in an altered way, or they may never be able to return to their pre-injury work.

Their new reality in a personal world is completely altered by an injury medical science persists in characterizing as "mild."

For some MTBI suffers, they may spend the rest of their lives faced with memory difficulties, problem solving, deductive reasoning, stress, cognitive fatigue, emotional control, depression, and frustration. They will certainly build a new "normal," but it will never be their old "normal."

Accepting that "new normal" is a crucial part of recovery. Otherwise, you will always be grappling with an inner battle that will prevent you from overcoming low moods and issues with self-esteem.

Chapter 6 – Finding What Works

The most difficult step all MTBI sufferers face is simply accepting and acknowledging that their brain has been damaged and that they may now be coping   with the fallout of that damage for life.

Using a word like "acceptance" can be both trite and facile without an acknowledgement of the magnitude of changes we are discussing. A person with MTBI has to in some way accept re-learning and monitoring their performance of tasks that were once so simple and automatic they required no thought whatsoever.

Many of these functions are "executive" in nature because they are integral to the day-to-day flow of life. Being aware of the day of the week and month doesn't just orient you chronologically, but is a factor of ordering your life, paying your bills, meeting deadlines associated with work, even getting a book back to the library on time.

Processing Speed Batters the Self-Esteem

When a person experiences a reduction in their ability to process and act upon information, the concurrent level of frustration is overwhelming and batters the self-esteem. Suddenly the world just moves too fast! You can't keep up and it's natural to tell yourself you're "stupid" (and quite often to lash out in anger because you just feel so awful physically and emotionally.)

It is imperative to let yourself off that hook. You are suffering from a brain injury that is less characterized by a visible wound and more by a disruption in the brain's metabolism.

Your brain has suffered shearing, twisting, and tearing forces that have stretched it out of shape. The cells are not functioning as they normally would.

Brain injury is not a commentary on your intelligence. To suggest that is the fact makes no more sense than saying, "He has a broken leg so he was never a good runner."

You must, however, follow the "logic" to the next stage. "He" may well be an exceptional runner, but because he broke his leg, he won't run the same way in the future.

After an MTBI you may not think the same way, but you will think – effectively and efficiently – just according to new paradigms that you will create to fit your altered way of being in the world.

The Effects of Slower Processing

Some of the most common manifestations of slower processing speed include things like:

- An inability to hold more than one thought at a time.
- Getting lost in a conversation.
- Not "getting" jokes.
- Being unable to follow plots.
- Forgetting why you've walked into a room.
- Letting your sentences go unfinished.
- Being unable to pick up on non-verbal cues.

An even more serious complication can be an inability to judge the consequences of an action. The instructions on a frozen dinner might read, "Cook in a 450 degree F oven for

30 minutes." They do not say, "Take the dinner out of the cardboard box and then put the tray in a 450 degree F oven."

Someone with MTBI might not pick up on this fact and put the entire box in the oven without realizing the cardboard will catch on fire.

Overall Coping Mechanisms

Working with rehabilitation professionals, you will develop individualized coping mechanisms for your specific issues. There are, however, a number of general-purpose strategies that will help to mitigate the often interlocking and cascading effects of MTBI.

Managing Your Environment

Becoming overwhelmed by stimuli is a major hurdle MTBI patients face daily. As you work to regain control of your executive thinking, simply creating an atmosphere in which you can focus is essential – both at home and at work.

Making changes to your environment may be as minor as turning the TV off while you pay the bills, or asking your boss to move your desk out of a busy hive of cubicles and into an area with fewer distractions.

Don't be reluctant to ask for the accommodations you need to function. You have legal rights in the workplace. In the United States, people with MTBI enjoy the protection of The Americans with Disabilities Act, while those in the United Kingdom are covered by the Equality Act 2010.

If you discuss your problems with your employer and explain the need for your work area to be changed, compliance with that request is legally mandated.

Seek Out Quiet Time

Whether you are at home or at work, understand the value of quiet time in regaining your equilibrium and focus. When you begin to feel overwhelmed, your organizational skills will deteriorate rapidly and you may begin to panic.

In those moments, you need to get to some place quiet so you can calm down and regroup. Do not, however, just reserve quiet times for emergency situations. Use quiet moments in the day as a way to prevent becoming over-stressed.

Go to the park during lunch, sit quietly for a few minutes in a church or library, or listen to something soothing through your headphones. "Time outs" prevent your brain from hitting overload and really shutting down.

This may include getting a nap in when you feel like you need one. The fatigue of working so hard to concentrate and staying on track can be crushing.

The more tired you become, the less able you are to function and to manage your emotional responses. A "power nap" can work wonders in "rebooting" your brain.

Kindly Watch the Clock

It's important to consciously re-cultivate your awareness of time, but not to pit yourself against the clock. See time for what it is – a tool. Obviously the clock is essential to help you keep appointments and order your day, but it's also a vital measurement device.

For a person with MTBI, budgeting time is extremely important since the negative effects of feeling rushed can be disastrous. Some MTBI sufferers become almost paralyzed when they're pushed to meet deadlines. Your goal is to find out how long it takes you to complete everyday tasks and to make sure you have that amount of time to move at your own pace.

It doesn't matter if you "used" to be ready for work in half an hour. In the aftermath of your MTBI, you may need an hour or more.

Find out what the real number is and work with it. Better to take longer and arrive at work on time and in a good frame of mind to start the day, rather than push yourself and be flustered and overwhelmed before the workday has even started.

You may need to elicit the help of a loved one or friend to get the accurate information you need to really work out a time budget.

We all tend to over-estimate our abilities, but MTBI patients can be so determined to look and act "normal" that they are not at all realistic about scheduling.

Don't just work with "guess-timates." Create an actual, workable, daily schedule based on real benchmarks.

Be flexible. If a new task comes into your life, budget more time than you think you need to learn what you're doing. Continue to monitor the time required to complete the task until you feel you've hit your comfortable pace.

Find Good Coping Tools and Use Them

Don't regard coping devices as crutches - see them as tools. For instance, put a voice recording application on your cell phone or acquire a small stand-alone recording device.

When you park in a large lot, describe where you're parked in a way you will understand it when you play it back. Alternatively try and park in the same place each time.

Work on including the relevant information.

Saying, "I'm parked on the third row from the street between a red truck and a blue van," won't get the job done, although that might be exactly the way a person with MTBI would interpret the situation, failing to realise that those vehicles might not be there when they come back.

Instead say, "I'm parked in the third row from the street in space M3. Look at the ceiling above the cars. That's where the numbers are painted."

This version not only gives the specific location of the car according to a fixed standard, but it helps you remember where to locate that fixed standard.

Recording information in this manner, whether by voice or by jotting a note, will not only help you to retain the specific data you need, but it will also serve as practice for being in the world with more of the focused attention you've lost due to your injury.

You may also want to:

- Make a list for your day-to-day routine. This can be invaluable to helping you get a handle on what you need to accomplish on any given day. Have a checklist and keep a routine that works for you.

- Pre-plan. For instance, if you are traveling, note the routes and the major landmarks. This will prevent panic if you suddenly have the feeling that something is just not right.

- Organize your home and work environment so things are always in the same place, especially the things you use every day, like car keys, handbags, or briefcases.

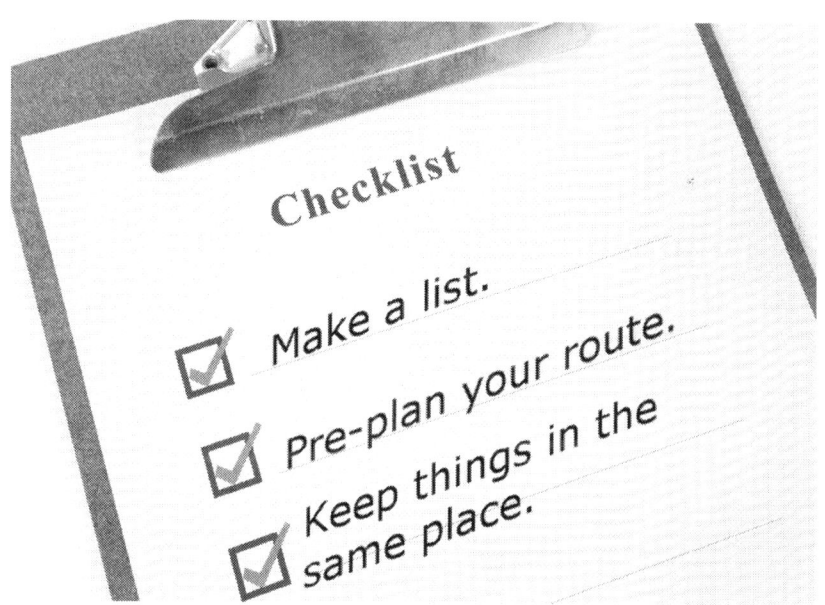

Creating a Climate for Recovery

Using general-purpose coping strategies helps to create a climate for recovery that will better accommodate all the individualized things you may need to do to live with your unique case of MTBI. Brain injuries are like fingerprints.

No two cases are the same, and even two people who were injured at the same time, in the same way, in the same accident will not exhibit the same MTBI symptoms.

Afterword

In the Foreword, I stated my purpose as a desire to equip readers with enough information to ask better questions and to seek better answers. Now, my hope is that you will be well enough informed to interpret those answers in the context of your life or that of your loved one.

Mild traumatic brain injury does not happen to individuals in isolation. For all that the injured person suffers in terms of cognitive and functional deficits, their friends and family are suddenly confronted with a person who looks exactly like the loved one they've always known, but who may act in ways that are bewildering.

The wars in Iraq and Afghanistan vaulted traumatic brain injury into the public limelight, as did the injuries suffered by ABC anchorman Bob Woodward and Arizona Congresswoman Gabrielle Giffords. The dangers of MTBI however, and its signature injury, concussion, have come into our awareness by a more potentially chilling venue – the sports field.

Professional athletes suffering early onset dementia as a consequence of repeated concussions are tragic, but these are grown men who made their own choices.

The fact that the beginning signs of the same disease were found during the autopsy of an 18-year-old multi-sport high school athlete is a parent's worst nightmare. Had this young man lived, he would have begun to experience the symptoms of dementia in his early 50s. Could this have been prevented? In all likelihood, yes, but by a route that a sports-obsessed culture finds difficult to stomach – time on the bench.

In Europe blood tests are routinely used to detect the presence of a key protein that should be found only in the brain. If it is in the blood, the chemical has crossed the blood / brain barrier and brain injury is present. Such a benchmark gives doctors a definitive point of argument to say, "Your child has suffered a concussion and can't play sports until he/she has sufficiently recovered."

In the United States, however, young athletes readily admit that although they are aware of the long-term dangers of concussion, they have or would lie about their medical condition to get back on the playing field.

For anyone who has suffered an MTBI from any source, this sounds like what it is, utter madness. Far from being just a case of getting "clocked" or "having your bell rung," MTBI is a life-altering event. Some people heal with seemingly no after affects; others grapple with life-long deficits. They do recover, but not with the same abilities they had before they were hurt.

Ninety percent of MTBIs are caused by concussion. It is imperative that those who suffer from an MTBI, their family and friends, and society as a whole understand the severity of this silent epidemic, and direct research dollars to better prevention and enhanced treatment options.

There is nothing mild about mild traumatic brain injury. Some 2.5 million people in the United States and Europe suffer these injuries on an annual basis.

Many MTBIs are preventable, and all are treatable. Brain injury is not something to hide or something over which you should suffer shame. It is a wound, a largely invisible one in terms of sutures and scars, but just as serious as any traumatic injury in terms of pain and frustration.

By bringing this subject fully into the light and understanding all the components of MTBI, a truly proactive healing can begin.

Frequently Asked Questions

Brain injury is a broad topic and a highly individualized experience. Some of the more common questions asked include the following, but to get a more complete picture of MTBI, its causes, effects, and long-term consequences, please refer to the full text.

How do brain injuries generally happen?

Accidents or assaults are the most frequent cause of brain injury, which may also happen when the oxygen supply to the brain is diminished or cut off by a stroke or even an infection.

Closed brain injuries happen when the brain hits another surface and is jarred severely. An open brain injury is the result of the brain being penetrated.

The vast majority of instances of mild traumatic brain injury (MTBI) are the result of a concussion, a jarring of the brain that may not even cause a loss of consciousness. In these cases, symptoms may not surface for a number of hours or even days.

What do doctors do to determine how severe a brain injury is?

Rating the severity of brain injury is actually more imprecise than you might think, especially where MTBI is concerned. The accepted levels of severity are: mild, moderate, and severe.

Some of the common measurement scales used to assess brain injury are discussed in Chapter 2, including the Glasgow Coma Scale and the Rancho Los Amigos Scale.

How do acquired brain injuries differ from traumatic brain injuries?

Traumatic brain injuries are caused by external forces like automobile accidents, physical assaults, falls, or even gunshot wounds.

Acquired brain injuries include strokes (cerebral vascular accidents) and oxygen deprivation (hypoxic brain injury.)

Other injuries to the brain that are progressive include, but are not limited to Parkinson's or Alzheimer's disease.

All levels of brain injuries cause some degree of disruption in the brain function, on a scale from mild to severe.

What are anoxic and hypoxic brain injuries?

Anoxic brain injury refers to the brain being completely deprived of oxygen, whereas hypoxic is insufficient oxygen for an extended period of time.

In the absence of oxygen, brain cells die. The more cells that are compromised, the more brain function is impaired.

Some common causes of both anoxic and hypoxic brain injury include:
- Drowning or near drowning.
- Electrical shock.
- Heart attack or other coronary episodes.
- Brain tumour.
- Choking, both intentional and accidental.
- Poisoning, particularly from carbon monoxide.
- Suffocation, both intentional and accidental.

What are neuropsychologists and what do they do?

Neuropsychologists evaluate the specific problems a patient is experiencing, evaluating their overall issues, and arriving at a plan for optimum progress in rehabilitation. As such, they are crucial members of an individual's rehabilitation team, and may also act as counsellors.

What are cognitive problems and what kind may be present?

Any deficit in skill following a brain injury may be classed as a cognitive problem. These might include issues with:

- Becoming over-stimulated by things in the surrounding environment, or even by complex questions or tasks.

- Attention deficits and an inability to filter out some sensory stimuli like sound or light.

- Short-term memory problems.

- Difficulty acquiring new information and learning.

- Higher level thinking, often referred to as "executive" skills.

- Carrying a conversation for an extended period of time or following a group conversation without experiencing intense fatigue.

Some cognitive issues resolve over time or improve as coping skills develop, but others persist or become permanent, often contributing to "neurobehavioral" problems.

What is a "neurobehavioral" problem?

Any problem that can be tied to a specific aspect of a brain injury is described as "neurobehavioral." This may be a loss of normal inhibitions so that the person is not able to self-regulate for appropriate speech, or may have difficulty controlling anger and expressions of frustration. Impaired judgment is also a factor and over-reactions are typical

Medications may assist with controlling unacceptable behaviours, but more often, in consult with a neuropsychologist, strategies are put in place for the patient to re-learn what is and is not acceptable, as well as how to recognize and avoid triggers in their lives.

Why do people with brain injuries have anger control issues?

Sometimes the anger issues are simply born of the frustration the person feels due to cognitive stress and an inability to filter a flood of information. At other times, however, anger issues are directly linked to injuries in the frontal lobe of the brain, the part of the organ most responsible for regulating impulse control.

Why is it difficult for people with brain injury to control their emotions?

Again, issues with emotions often stem from frustration. It is typical, however, with cases of MTBI, especially in the presence of concussion, for the patient to experience extreme sadness to the point of grief and profound depression.

The person may burst into tears not only because they are unable to perform a task or answer a question, but also because they are dealing with such deep feelings of sadness.

Can you explain mild brain injury?

Another term for mild brain injury is "subtle acquired brain injury." For the people who are coping with the cognitive, psychological and physical fallout of MTBI, however, their condition does not feel subtle or mild.

In medical terms, however, the initial injury did not lead to a long period of unconsciousness. In fact, the person may not have lost consciousness at all, and their symptoms may have presented slowly over a period of hours or days.

Until recently, it was not clearly understood that the effects of MTBI do not resolve in 2-3 weeks as previously thought, but can permanently change the person's ability to think and function.

Are there physical symptoms with MTBI?

Yes, there are a wide range of physical symptoms including, but not limited to:

- Dizziness and / or vertigo.
- Motion sickness.
- Nausea.
- Persistent fatigue.
- Tinnitus or "ringing" in the ears.
- Persistent and recurring headaches.
- Sensitivity (often hypersensitivity) to touch, tastes, smells, sounds, and noises.
- Sensitivity to busy, crowded environments.
- Sensitivity to unfamiliar places, persons, and circumstances.

What are the psychological and emotional problems associated with MTBI?

The psychological and emotional problems present with MTBI are often significant enough that other people say the person has a "changed personality." These things may include:

- Anxiety.
- Depression.
- Not sleeping enough, or sleeping too much.
- Decreased (or increased) sex drive.
- Fearfulness.
- Temperament changes (often with anger control issues.)
- Lack of self-esteem and confidence.

Poor judgment, especially as related to impulse control can also contribute to psychological and emotional issues if the use of drugs or alcohol are part of the equation.

Do people with MTBI have actual psychiatric problems?

Many people who experience an MTBI do wind up under the care of a psychiatrist or psychologist. This is due in part to their often extreme emotional reactions to triggering stimuli.

Depending on the manner in which the person was initially injured, it is possible to suffer from Post-Traumatic Stress Disorder (PTSD) in addition to the brain injury itself.

How do MTBI symptoms emerge? How long does it take?

It's quite common for there to be two sets of symptoms with MTBI, those that occur just after the incident itself, and those that present within a few hours or days.

The initial symptoms generally include some mix of:

- Headaches
- Nausea
- Dizziness
- Confusion
- Agitation
- Disorientation
- Amnesia
- Fatigue

(Note that fatigue and headache can become persistent for months.)

The next layer of symptoms may not surface until the person has "recovered" for two or three weeks and tries to go back to their normal level of activities. This is when they realise they have functional impairments affecting cognition, emotions, and even physical abilities like balance.

It is this stage that is often most difficult for the MTBI patient to manage because they have not yet accepted that they are injured with long-term consequences.

Is a concussion a mild brain injury?

Concussion is actually the most common form of MTBI, and is responsible for 75% to 90% of all reported cases. Until the last five years, concussion was thought to be a temporary injury.

The most recent research has shown, however, that when the nerve fibres in the brain are stretched or torn by a concussion the effects can be long term.

Concussive injuries don't show up on conventional neurological scans like CAT or MRI. If the patient did not lose consciousness in the accident, there may, in fact, be no initial neurological exam.

Often concussions are not diagnosed until the patient complains of the cascade of physical, emotional, and cognitive symptoms typically referred to as Post-Concussion Syndrome (PCS).

Are there serious effects from repeated concussions while playing sports?

Repeated concussions are a very serious problem because the effects are cumulative and have been conclusively linked with early onset dementia caused by chronic traumatic encephalopathy (CTE), a disease that presents in much the same way as Alzheimer's.

Recent findings of CTE in professional football players has led to a push for increased awareness of the danger of concussion injuries in young athletes.

To date, the youngest individual whose brain tested positive for CTE was an 18-year-old multi-sports athlete killed in an accident. Had the boy lived, he would have suffered from early onset dementia in his 50s, due to the repeated concussions he suffered playing football in high school.

How do people with MTBI act right after the accident?

People with MTBI will often say they feel depressed or feel like they're losing their minds. They will have great difficulty understanding and accepting what is happening to them, and will fight persistent headaches and fatigue. They will also grapple with:

- Mood swings
- Angry outbursts
- Poor concentration
- Insomnia
- Poor appetite
- Confusion

Often the very professionals to whom these people turn for help do not themselves understand MTBI and offer very little relief, and at times, are not even sympathetic or empathetic.

Can someone "fake" MTBI?

It would be extremely difficult to consistently maintain the pattern of cognitive and emotional deficits present in MTBI. However, because the person "looks" okay, it is quite common for someone with a brain injury to be accused of "malingering" or manufacturing their condition to get off work.

There are numerous assessment tools to prove this is not the case, but the person with the injury may grapple with feelings of guilt for not getting well fast enough or for their inability to function at their pre-injury level both at home and at work.

Will rehab programs help someone recover from MTBI?

Rehabilitation is crucial to recovering from MTBI because it is in the safe environment of therapy that the patient can develop coping strategies to deal with their deficits.

Additionally, the counselling services available to them and to their loved ones are invaluable in creating a broader foundation for their long-term recovery and improvement.

When can someone with MTBI go back to work?

Resuming work or career-related activities are an important part of rehabilitation from MTBI. People who try to go back to work after such an injury, without having professional help, will experience the greatest range of problems, often suffering in silence for fear that they will lose their position if they say anything.

Each case is unique, both in terms of the individual and of their employment. Effective rehabilitation programs include a component for transition of the person back to their job at a level they can handle proportionately handle with their current level of recovery.

If this is not possible, the individual may need to consider a different vocation more suited to their changed emotional and physical abilities and mental stamina.

How can friends and family help someone suffering from MTBI?

Education is essential to understand what your loved one is going through. Be a part of the rehabilitation team by finding out from the therapists and professionals involved exactly what you can do to help in ways both practical and emotional.

At the same time, however, take care of yourself. You need your rest, and you may well need to seek the aid of a professional counsellor to deal with your own anger and frustration over the changes in your loved one that have altered the quality of your life.

Venting those feelings toward your loved one will only introduce tension into the situation, this is counter-productive to both your relationship with that person and for their long-term recovery prospects. At the same time, however, failing to honour your own feelings is not healthy for you.

Relevant Websites

American Association of Nurse Life Care Planners
http://www.aanlcp.org/

American Brain Coalition
http://www.americanbraincoalition.org/

American Congress of Rehabilitation Medicine
http://www.acrm.org/

American Occupational Therapy Association, Inc.
http://www.aota.org/

American Physical Therapy Association
http://www.apta.org/

American Speech-Language-Hearing Association
http://www.asha.org/public/

Australasian Society for the Study of Brain Impairment
http://www.assbi.com.au/

Brain Injury Association of America
http://www.biausa.org/

Brain Injury Association of Canada
http://biac-aclc.ca/

Brain Injury Australia
http://www.braininjuryaustralia.org.au/
Brain Trauma Foundation
https://www.braintrauma.org/

Canadian Association of Neuroscience Nurses
http://www.cann.ca/

Commission on Accreditation of Rehabilitation Facilities
http://www.carf.org/home/

Encephalitis Society
http://www.encephalitis.info/

Euroacademia Multidisciplinaria Neurotraumatologica
http://www.emn.cc/start.htm

European Brain Injury Society
http://www.ebissociety.org/

European Neurological Society
http://www.ensinfo.org/

Foundation for Life Care Planning Research, Inc.
http://www.flcpr.org/

International Association of Rehabilitation Professionals
http://www.rehabpro.org/

International Pediatric Brain Injury Society
http://www.ipbis.org/

Latin American Brain Injury Consortium
http://www.internationalbrain.org/articles/latin-american-brain-injury-consortium-labic/

North American Brain Injury Society
http://www.nabis.org/

Sarah Jane Brain Foundation
http://www.thebrainproject.org/

Society for Cognitive Rehabilitation
http://www.societyforcognitiverehab.org/

Society for Research in Rehabilitation
http://www.srr.org.uk/

World Federation for NeuroRehabilitation
http://wfnr.co.uk/

Brain Injury Rehabilitation Resources - US

Source: Brain Injury Resources at
www.headinjry.com/rehabfacility.htm

Arizona

Good Samaritan Regional Medical Centre
1111 East McDowell Road
Phoenix, AZ 85006
Tel. 602-239-2000

California

CareMeridian
18 A Journey, Ste. #200
Aliso Viejo, CA 92656
Tel. 949-263-6630 Ext. 1116
www.caremeridian.com

Casa Colina Centres for Rehabilitation
255 East Bonita Ave
Pomona, CA 91769-6001
Tel. 909-596 7733 Ext 2221
Toll Free: 800-926-5462
FAX 909-593 0153

www.casacolina.org

Cedars-Sinai Medical Centre

8700 Beverly Blvd,

Los Angeles, CA 90048

Tel. 310-855-5000

Childrens Hospital

4650 Sunset Blvd.

Los Angeles, CA 90027

Tel. 323- 660-2450

Good Samaritan Hospital

616 South Witmer Street

Los Angeles, CA 90017

The Health Restoration Medical Centre

26381 Crown Valley #130

Mission Viejo, CA 92691

Tel. 949-367-8870

Toll Free: 800- 300-1063

FAX: (949) 367-9779

www.strokedoctor.com/map.htm

Loma Linda University Medical Centre

11234 Anderson Street

Loma Linda, CA 92354

Long Beach Memorial Medical Centre

2801 Atlantic Avenue

Long Beach, CA 90806

Colorado

Boulder Community Hosp. Mapleton Rehab Ctr

311 Mapleton Ave.

Boulder CO 80301-9130

303-441-0537

Children's Hospital

1056 East 19th Avenue

Denver, CO 80218

Tel. 303-861-6730

www.thechildrenshospital.org/index.cfm

Craig Hospital, Englewood

3425 South Clarkson

Englewood, CO 80110

Tel: 303-789-8000

www.craighospital.org

Florida

Bayfront Medical Centre

9700 9th Street North, Suite 300

St. Petersburg, FL 33702

Tel. 727-579-8077;

FAX: 727-577-7594

Bayview Neurohealth and Quality Living, Inc.

325 Braden Ave.

Sarasota, FL 34243

888-41-REHAB

www.bayviewneuro.com

Brain Injury Rehab Centre at Sand Lake Hospital (BIRC)

9400 Turkey Lake RD

Orlando FL 32819

Tel. 407-351-8538

FAX: 407-351-8584

Georgia

Emory University Hospital

1364 Clifton Rd NE

Atlanta, GA 30322

Tel. 404-778-7744

Illinois

Children's Memorial Hospital
2300 Children's Plaza
Chicago, IL 60614
Tel. 800-KIDS-DOC-
www.childrensmemorial.org

Cook County Hospital
1835 West Harrison Street
Chicago, IL 60612

Evanston Hospital
2650 Ridge Avenue
Evanston, IL 60201

F.G. McGaw Hospital at Loyola University
2160 South First Avenue
Maywood, IL 60153

Marianjoy Inc.
26W171 Roosevelt Rd.
Wheaton, IL 60187
Tel. 630-462-4204
FAX: 630-462-4440 --
www.marianjoy.org

Northwestern Memorial Hospital

250 East Superior Street

Chicago, IL 60611

Indiana

Indiana University Medical Centre

550 North University Boulevard

Indianapolis, IN 46202

Kansas

C. F. Menninger Memorial Hospital

5800 West Sixth Avenue

Topeka, KS 66606

Tel. 785-350-5553

Toll Free: 800-351-9058

Maryland

Bryn Mawr Rehab Centre - Maryland General

827 Linden Ave,

Baltimore, MD 21201

Tel. 410-2555-8522;

Toll Free: 800-410-8765

Greater Baltimore Medical Centre

6701 North Charles Street

Baltimore, MD 21204

Tel. 410-828-2000

Johns Hopkins Hospital

600 North Wolfe St.

Baltimore, MD 21287

Massachusetts

Berkshire Medical Centre

725 North St, Pittsfield, MA 01201,

413- 447-2200

Beth Israel Deaconess Medical

330 Brookline Ave, Boston, MA 02215

617- 667-3090

Boston Medical Centre

One Boston Medical Centre Place

Boston, MA 02118

Tel. 617-638-7300

FAX: 617-638-7313

Braintree Hospital Rehabilitation Network – TBI

250 Pond St, Braintree, MA 02185-9020

Tel. 617-848-5353 Ext. 2329;

Toll Free: 800-997-3422

FAX: 617-849-9949

Brigham and Women's Hospital

75 Francis Street, Boston, MA 02115

Tel. 617-732-5500

Toll Free: 800-722-5520

Children's Hospital

300 Longwood Avenue

Boston, MA 02115

Tel. 617- 355-6000

www.childrenshospital.org

Fairlawn Rehabilitation Hospital

189 May St.

Worcester, MA   01602

Tel. 508-791-6351

Toll Free: 800-442-1771

Greenery Rehabilitation Centre

23 Isaac St.

Middleboro, MA 02346

Tel. 508-947-9295

Ivy Street School

200 Ivy Street

Brookline, MA 02146

Telephone: 617-738-5116

Toll Free: 800-682-9200

Lahey Clinic

41 Mall Road

Burlington, MA 01805

New England Medical Centre

750 Washington Street

Boston, MA 02111

Michigan

Henry Ford Hospital

2799 West Grand Blvd.

Detroit, MI 48202

Tel. 313-876-2600

Toll Free: 800-653-6568

Hope Network Rehabilitation Services

Grand Rapids, Lansing, and Big Rapids, Michigan

www.hopenetworkrehab.org

Tel. 616-940-0040 Ext. 222

Minnesota

Bethesda Rehab Hospital

559 Capitol Blvd.

St. Paul, MN 55103

Courage Centre

3915 Golden Valley Road

Minneapolis, MN 55422

Tel. 763-520-0327

Gentiva Health Service - Rehab Without Walls

780 W. Lake Lansing Rd., Suite 200

East Lansing, MI 48823

Tel. 888-619-9735

FAX: 517-337-8467

www.gentiva.com/rehab_without_walls/

Hennepin County Medical Centre

701 Park Avenue South

Minneapolis, MN 55415

Tel. 612-347-2121

Mayo Clinic, Rochester

1216 Second Street SW

Rochester, MN 55902

Missouri

Barnes-Jewish Hospital

216 S Kingshighway Blvd.

Saint Louis, MO 63110

Tel. 314-747-3000

FAX: 314-362-8877

New Hampshire

Lakeview NeuroRehab Centre

101 Highwatch Road

Effingham Falls, NH 03814

Toll Free: 800- 473-4221

FAX: 603-539-8888

www.lakeviewsystem.com

Mary Hitchcock Memorial Hospital
One Medical Centre Drive
Lebanon, NH 03756

North Country Independent Living
1267 Village Square - PO Box 518
North Conway, NH 03860-0518
Tel. 603- 356-0282
Toll Free: 888-400-6245 (NCIL)
www.ncil4rehab.com

New Jersey

Atlantic Rehabilitation Institute
95 Mt. Kemble Ave.
Morristown, NJ 07960

Kessler Institute For Rehabilitation
1199 Pleasant Valley Way
West Orange, NJ 07052
www.kessler-rehab.com
www.rehabtrials.org

Mentor Network
505 South Lenola Road

Blason Office Plaza II, Suite 217

Moorestown, NJ 08057

Tel. 856-235-5505

FAX: 856-235-5506

New York

Brady Institute for Traumatic Brain Injury

8900 Van Wyck Expressway

Jamaica, New York 11418

718 206-7152

www.jamaicahospital.org

Burke Rehabilitation Hospital

785 Mamaroneck Ave.

White Plains, NY 10605

Tel. 914-597-2500

Toll Free: 888-99BURKE

burke.org/home.cfm

Columbia-Presbyterian Medical Centre

622 West 168th Street

New York, NY 10032

Tel. 212-305-2500 --

Toll Free: 800-227-CPMC

Helen Hayes Hospital Transitional Rehab Centre

80 Chapel Street

Garnerville, NY 10923

Hospital for Joint Diseases-Orthopedic Institute

301 East 17th Street,

New York, NY 10003

Hospital for Special Surgery

535 East 70th St.

New York, NY 10021

Long Island Jewish Medical Centre

27005 76th Avenue

New Hyde Park , NY 11040

New York Hospital-Cornell Medical Centre

525 East 68th Street

New York, NY 10021

Jamaica Hospital Medical Centre

8900 Van Wyck Expressway,

Jamaica, New York 11418 --

Tel. 718-206-6000

FAX: 718-206-6071

www.jamaicahospital.org

Mount Sinai Medical Centre
One Gustave L Levy Place
New York, NY 10029

North Carolina

Duke University Medical Centre
Erwin Road
Durham, NC 27710
Tel. 919-684-8111

North Carolina Baptist Hospital
Medical Centre Boulevard
Winston-Salem , NC 27157

Ohio

Children's Hospital Medical Centre
3333 Burnet Avenue
Cincinnati, OH 45229
Tel. 800-344-CHMC

Cleveland Clinic

9500 Euclid Avenue

Cleveland, OH 44195

Tel. 216-444-2200

Toll Free: 800-223-2273, Ext. 48950

Oklahoma

Brookhaven Hospital-- Neurologic Rehabilitation Institute (NRI)

201 S. Garnett Rd.

Tulsa, Oklahoma 74128-1800

Toll Free: 888-298-HOPE

Tel. 918-438-4257

www.brookhavenhospital.com

Oregon

Northwest Occupational Medical Centre, TBI Program

15862 SW 72 Ave

Portland OR 97224

Tel. 503-624-7246

FAX: 503-624-0724

Pennsylvania

Albert Einstein Medical Centre - Moss Rehabilitation Hospital
1200 West Tabor Road, Phila, PA
1-800-CALL-MOSS

Allegheny General Hospital
320 East North Ave, Pittsburgh, PA 15212
412-359-6200

Bryn Mawr Rehab Hospital
414 Paoli Pike, P.O. Box 3007
Malvern, PA 19355-3300
Tel. 610-251-5400
Toll Free: 888-REHAB-41
www.BrynMawrRehab.org

Children's Hospital of Philadelphia
34th St & Civic Centre Blvd
Philadelphia, PA 19104
Tel. 215-590-1000

Children's Hospital of Pittsburgh
3705 Fifth Avenue
Pittsburgh, PA 15213

Tel. 412-692-7240

www.chp.edu

Community Skills Program Counseling & Rehab

1500 Locus St. #1505

Philadelphia, PA 19102

Tel. 215-735-7603

FAX: 215-893-0502

HealthSouth Harmarville Rehabilitation Hospital

PO Box 11460 Guys Run Rd.

Pittsburgh, PA 15238

Tel. 412-826-2707

FAX: 412-828-1345

Hospital of the University of Pennsylvania

3400 Spruce Street

Philadelphia, PA 19104

Tel. 1-800-789-PENN (7366)

pennhealth.com/neuro/services/head_injury.html

Lehigh Valley Hospital,

Cedar Crest Blvd & I-78

Allentown, PA 18103

Magee Rehabilitation Hospital

Six Franklin Plaza

Philadelphia, PA 19102

Tel: 215-587-3000

Toll Free: 800-966-2433

FAX: 215-977-9740

Moss Rehabilitation Hospital

Moss Plaza, 9892 Bustleton Avenue

Philadelphia, PA

Toll Free: 800-CALL-MOSS

South Dakota

Community Transitions

1636 Concourse Ct.

Rapid City, SD 57703

Tel. 605-343-7297

Fax: 605-343-9309

www.brainrehab.org

Texas

Brown-Karhan Healthcare, Inc.

PO Box 419

Dripping Springs, TX 78620

Tel. 512-894-0701

www.brown-karhan.com

Centre For Neuro Skills - CNS Texas

3501 N. MacArthur Bldg 200

Irving, Texas 75062

Toll Free: 800-554-5448

Tel. 972-580-8500

Hermann Hospital

6411 Fannin

Houston, TX 77030

Tel. 704-4000

Neurobehavioral Resources, LTD

PO Box 929

Conroe, TX 77305-0929

Toll Free: 800-414-4TBI

Tel. 409-788-7785

Neurocognitive Rehabilitation Centre

1401 S. 2nd Ave.

Edinburg, TX 78539

Tel. 956-380-6550.

www.neurorehabcenter.com

Virginia

Concussion Care Centre of Virginia, Ltd.

10120 West Broad St., Suite G

Glen Allen, VA 23060

Tel. 804-270-5484;

www.cccv-ltd.com

Fairfax Hospital

3300 Gallows Road

Falls Church, VA 22046

Tel. 703-698-1110

John Jane Brain Injury Centre

534C East Main Street

Charlottesville, VA 22902

Tel. 434-220-3494

www.jjbic.org

Medical College of Virginia Hospitals

401 North 12th Street

Richmond, VA 23219

Tel. 804- 828-6284

Toll Free: 800-762-6161.

Washington

Centre for Medical Rehabilitation - Northwest Hospital & Medical
Centre
1550 N. 115th ST.
Seattle, WA 98133
Tel. 206-368-1794
FAX: 206-368-1399
www.nwhospital.org/services/rehab_main.asp

Children's Hospital and Medical Centre
4800 Sand Point Way NE
Seattle, WA 98105
Tel. 206-526-2000 -
Toll Free: 877-526-2500

Evergreen Head Injury Re-Entry Centre
12039 NE 128th St
Kirkland, WA 98034
Tel. 425-899-3100

Good Samaritan Medical Centre
407 14th Ave. SE
Puyallup, WA 98372
Tel. 253-697-4000
www.goodsamhealth.org

Washington, D.C.

Children's National Medical Centre
111 Michigan Avenue NW
Washington, DC 20010
Toll Free: 888-884-BEAR (2327)
Tel. 202-884-5000

Georgetown University Hospital
3800 Reservoir Road NW
Washington, DC 20007
Tel. 202-687-4355

National Rehabilitation Hospital
102 Irving Street NW
Washington, DC 20010

Brain Injury Rehabilitation Resources - UK

References

Headway Brain Trauma Booklets

Headway – the national brain injury association for the UK. The national contact will have a directory of local groups. National Helpline no is 0808-8002244. The Brain Injury Association in UK. www.headway.org.uk

Rehabilitation

www.ucl.ac.uk/ion/nationalhospital   is the national hospital specialising in neurologically and neuroscience. To see a specialist you will need a General Practioner referral (GP referral whether this is under the NHS or privately)

The Oxford Centre of Enablement http://www.ouh.nhs.uk

UKABIF UK – Acquired Brain Injury Forum – directory of rehabilitation services for ABI within the UK (2005) www.ukabif.org.uk

Rehabilitation for younger adults http://qef.org.uk/our-services/neuro-rehabilitation-services/

Communication difficulties

Connect is a charity for supporting People with Aphasia –

www.ukconnect.org

www.aphasiahelp.org

www.speakability.org.uk

Royal College of Speech and Language Therapists 020 7378 1200

www.rcslt.org

Sexual Functioning

To find a relationship and psychosexual therapist

www.relate.org.uk   www.basrt.org.uk

For PTSD and emotional trauma support and therapy

Lists of accredited counsellors and psychologists within the UK

0870 4435252 www.babcp.org.uk

List of registered psychologists and neuropsychologists

http://www.bps.org.uk/psychology-public/find-psychologist/find-psychologist

Brain Injury Rehabilitation Additional Resources

New Zealand

Brain Injury Association of New Zealand www.brain-injury.org.nz

Australia

Brain Injury Association of Australia www.bia.net.au

Ireland

Irish National Association of Acquired Brain Injury

www.headway.ie

Canada

Brain Injury Association of Canada www.biac.acla.ca

International

International Brain Injury Association www.international-brain.org

Glossary

A

Abstract concept – Concepts or ideas that are abstract are not fixed. They can be applied to different objects and situations, and are thus difficult for people with MTBI to comprehend.

Abstract thinking – The ability to comprehend and to apply abstract concepts to appropriate situations and surroundings including those that are novel to the person's experience.

Acquired brain injury – The medical implication is that an individual with an acquired brain injury has exhibited normal function until the time of sustaining an injury to the brain, which then resulted in impaired brain function.

Adaptive equipment – Any device, which, in its purpose and function, aids in the performance of some aspect of work, leisure, self-care, or exercise. Normally used by people with some degree of disability.

Affect – The emotional condition of an individual at any moment in time, which can be discerned from observation of that person.

Agraphia – The inability in writing to express thoughts.

Alexia – The inability to read written words on the page.

Ambulate – The action of walking. (A person who can walk is described as being ambulatory.)

Amnesia – A condition in which an individual cannot summon any memory of events that occurred before a specific moment in time, or in proximity to that moment in time.

Anomia – An inability, even in the presence of fluent speech, to recall the names of common objects, which can otherwise be described correctly.

Anosmia – A loss of the ability to use the sense of smell.

Anoxia – Lack of oxygen to the brain, resulting in deprivation of the brain cells, with subsequent functional damage relative to the length of time oxygen was diminished or cut off.

Antidepressants – Any medication that is used for the purposes of relieving depression.

Aphasia – An inability, caused by brain damage or other damage to the organs of speech and hearing that leaves an individual unable to express oneself and/or to understand language.

Articulation – The correct movement and placement of the palate, tongue, lips, and teeth for the purposes of clear speech and correct pronunciation.

Assistive equipment – Devices or equipment that, by their design, are helpful in allowing an individual to independently engage in work, leisure, physical exercise, and self-care.

Attention – The capacity to focus on a task or stimuli for a length of time adequate for the task at hand, for instance the plot of a film, or the topic of a talk.

Audiologist – A professional who evaluates an individual to judge the degree of hearing defects present and then aids in correcting those defects with rehabilitation measures including electronic hearing aids.

B

Balance – The use of physical reactions to maintain an upright state with correct equilibrium, whether the position be standing or sitting.

Behaviour – The sum total of an individual's actions and reactions.

Behaviour disorders – Patterns of action and reaction that are in some way uncontrolled, inappropriate, dangerous, unacceptable, destructive, or counter-productive. The correction and amelioration of such behaviours is often a goal of rehabilitation.

Bilateral – Of or pertaining to both the left and right sides of something.

Brain plasticity – The ability of healthy, intact cells in the brain to take over and do the jobs once performed by damaged cells. Plasticity decreases as an individual ages.

Brain scan – Using radioactive dye injected into the blood stream, this imaging method is used to detect the presence of blood clots and haemorrhages, tumours, abscesses, and any anatomical abnormalities.

C

Case management – The procedure by which a patient's care is facilitated, often through a liaison, to coordinate the efforts of support and rehabilitation programs for the optimal delivery of services across multiple professional offices and agencies.

Cerebral-spinal fluid – The fluid that surrounds the spinal cord and is present around the brain and in the ventricles.

Chronic – Any condition marked by either frequent recurrence or a long duration of presence.

Closed brain injury – Brain injuries of this nature happen when the head first accelerates and then decelerates or slows down rapidly (or collides with an object.) The violent forces subject the delicate tissues of the brain to twisting, tearing, stretching, and smashing forces. The resulting disabilities tend to be highly variable and widely generalized.

Cognition – The process by which a person is conscious or aware of their own perceptions and thoughts and is capable of reasoning and understanding. Roughly synonymous with the word "thought."

Cognitive rehabilitation – Programs of therapy designed to aid a person in regaining their problem solving and thinking skills, including perception and memory. The work involves learning coping strategies and actively practicing skills with a goal of regaining and/or improving function of achieving compensation for deficits. Every program of cognitive rehabilitation is unique, based on assessment of the deficits present, and coordinated for optimal returns by qualified rehabilitation specialists.

Coma – Patients in a state of coma are so deeply unconscious they cannot be awakened by powerful stimulation. They do not respond to anyone or anything in their environment.

Communicative disorder – An impaired ability to process or receive input and concepts from a system of symbols, such as language, and to transmit and use those symbols in response.

Comprehension – The ability to understand communication received via the spoken or written word or by gestures.

Computerized axial tomography – In this diagnostic test, a series of x-rays are taken that visualize different levels of the brain, the skull, and other intracranial structures. Also referred to as a CAT or CT scan, this test is often used to determine the need for surgery, or as a means of measuring the degree of recovery after a brain injury.

Concentration – An individual's ability to focus for an appropriate amount of time on a given task or set of stimuli.

Concrete thinking – In this thinking mode, the individual views each situation with which he is presented as unique. There is no demonstrable ability to recognize and generalize similarities between situations. The perceptions and language used to describe what is going on are highly literal, and the patient cannot grasp the metaphorical meaning of statements like, "tight as bark on a tree."

Concussion – This injury represents 90 percent of all cases of mild traumatic brain injury and results from either a blow to the head or a sudden deceleration of the head. The result is a temporary or potentially prolonged altered mental state caused by the disruption of the physical integrity of the affected brain cells. May or may not be accompanied by a loss of consciousness.

Confabulation – The tendency of brain injury sufferers to create people, places, or events to fill gaps in their perception that have no basis in reality. The accounts may be highly detailed and delivered with tremendous conviction.

Confusion – A mental state in which an individual has no capacity to self-orient and is bewildered and perplexed by what is going on around them.

Contrecoup – Bruising on the brain that occurs on the opposite side of the brain from which the actual blow was delivered.

D

Diffuse axonal injury – One of the two apparently primary lesions present in brain injury. The other is haemorrhage, created by stretching or shearing of blood vessels. A diffuse axonal injury is a shearing injury of the large nerve fibres present in many areas of the brain.

Diffuse brain injury – Cell injuries in many areas of the brain rather than being confined to one specific location.

Disinhibition – An inability to inhibit or to suppress impulsive emotions or behaviours.

Disorientation – A state in which an individual does not know their identity or location, nor can they supply the current date. Medical professions refer to a normal state of orientation as "times three," aware of person, place, and time.

E

Electroencephalogram (EEG) – A procedure in which electrodes are attached to the scalp for the purpose of recording electrical brain activity to detect conditions like epilepsy, coma, and brain death.

Emotional lability – Rapid and drastic emotional changes for no apparent reason and often inappropriately, for instance swinging between hysterical laughter and sobbing.

Episodic memory – Refers to memories of ongoing life events. More easily disrupted than semantic memory because less rehearsal or repetition is present.

Extremity – In reference to the human body, either an arm or a leg.

F

Flaccid – Limp. Lacking in a normal degree of muscle tone.

Frustration tolerance – A person's ability to persist for the amount of time required to complete a task regardless of any apparent difficulties. A typical response of individual's with poor frustration tolerance is a refusal to complete any task with a perceived degree of difficulty. Indications of the level of frustration may include anger, yelling, and throwing of objects.

G

Glasgow Coma Scale – A standardized system that relies on eye opening, verbal responses, and motor responses as determinants for the evaluation of the degree of brain injury present.

H

Head injury – Any injury to the head or brain including lacerations and contusions as well as traumatic brain injuries and concussion (mild traumatic brain injury.)

Hypoxia – A condition in which an insufficient amount of oxygen reaches the body's tissues.

I

Immediate memory – The capacity to recall bits of information immediately after their presentation like words, numbers, and images. Individuals with immediate memory problems find learning new tasks difficult, as they cannot retain instructions.

Impulse control – The ability to hold back inappropriate physical and verbal responses during task completion. Not acting or speaking without first considering the consequences.

L

Lability – A state in which significant shifts in emotions occur, for instance wild laughter or uncontrollable weeping.

Long-term memory – The ability to recall information and to retrieve that information thirty minutes or more after its presentation.

M

Magnetic resonance imaging (MRI) – The use of electromagnetic energy for diagnostic purposes to generate images of the body's soft tissues, central nervous system, and skeleton.

N

Neuropsychologist – A psychologist specializing in the testing and evaluation of brain function as it relates to behaviour. Works with brain injury survivors to develop training programs geared toward restoring normal function, or the creation of alternative strategies that minimize the effect of the brain injury on daily life.

P

Perception – The ability to correctly interpret sensory input including sights, sounds, tastes, odours, and touches. In MTBI cases perceptual loss is often subtle.

Physiatrist – A physician specializing in physical medicine and rehabilitation including neurologic rehabilitation.

Physical therapist – A therapist trained to evaluate the potential for functional movement in an affected individual, who then develops a treatment program geared toward creating functional independence for the patient. Components of movement routinely evaluated by physical therapists include, but are not limited to muscle strength and tone, posture, coordination, endurance, and overall mobility.

Plasticity – The influence of ongoing activity on the function of cellular or tissue structures.

Plateau – A levelling off of progress in the process of recovery or rehabilitation that may be temporary or permanent.

Problem-solving skill – The ability to consider any relevant factors likely to influence the outcome of solutions to be applied to a given problem, and the subsequent ability to pick from those solutions the one that is most advantageous. MTBI patients often become paralyzed when confronted with multiple potential solutions to a problem because they lack these filtering skills.

Prognosis – Using the nature and symptoms of an injury or disease to predict the prospect for the patient's recovery.

Psychologist – Mental health professional specializing in counselling including the development of adjustment strategies and compensatory measures in cases of disability.

R

Rehabilitation – Any comprehensive program of a combination of mental, physical, and occupational therapies designed to reduce and overcome any deficits created by illness or injury.

Rehabilitation counsellor – Alternately called a vocational counsellor, these specialists' help patients develop aptitudes and skills necessary to return to a functional level of activity and productivity in the community.

Rehabilitation facility – Any coordinated service or services, offered by an agency to resident or non-resident patients for the purpose of minimizing or correcting physical, mental, or vocational difficulties resulting from disease or injury.

Rehabilitation nurse – Nurses trained in rehabilitation techniques who work in rehabilitation facilities both treating patients and working with their families to acquire the necessary skills and information for long-term functional recovery.

S

Sensation – Any stimuli which activates feelings in the body's sensory organs, for instance, touch, temperature, pressure, and/or pain

Short-term memory – The working memory of conscious awareness with a capacity to hold approximately seven chunks of information for a period of 30 seconds to several minutes depending on the attention being paid to the current task at hand.

T

Traumatic Brain Injury (TBI) – Damage to the living tissue of the human brain delivered by external, mechanical forces. TBIs are normally characterized by periods of altered consciousness including coma, or some degree of amnesia. Consequent disabling conditions may include, but are not limited to, orthopaedic, visual, aural, neurologic, perceptive/cognitive, or mental/emotional.

Sources Cited

Arciniegas, David B., C. Alan Anderson, and Thomas McAllister, "Mild Traumatic Brain Injury: A Neuropsychiatric Approach to Diagnosis, Evaluation, and Treatment," Neuropsychiatric Disease and Treatment, December 2005 (1:4) 311-327.

"Brain Injury Facts," International Brain Injury Association, http://www.internationalbrain.org/brain-injury-facts/ , Accessed June 2013.

Castillo, Michelle. "Most High School Football Players Would Still Play After Concussion." CBS News, 6 May 2013, http://www.cbsnews.com/8301-204_162-57583063/most-high-school-football-players-would-still-play-after-concussion/ (Accessed July 2013).

Dambinova, Svetlana A. "Diagnostic Challenges in Traumatic Brain Injury," IVD Technology, http://www.ivdtechnology.com/article/diagnostic-challenges-traumatic-brain-injury (Accessed July 2013).

Freeman, Mike. "Anniversary of Junior Seau Death Still Focuses NFL on CTE," CBS Sports, 2 May 2013, http://www.cbssports.com/nfl/blog/mike-freeman/22183367/anniversary-of-junior-seau-death-still-focuses-nfl-on-cte (Accessed July 2013).

Mangels, John. "Non-Concussion Football Head Hits Can Cause Brain Changes, Cleveland Clinic-Led Study Finds, Cleveland.com, http://www.cleveland.com/science/index.ssf/2013/03/non-concussion_football_head_h.html (Accessed July 2013).

Mann, Denise as reviewed by Louise Chang, MD. "Bob Woodruff After Traumatic Brain Injury: ABC News Journalist Bob Woodruff Talks About His Recovery From a Traumatic Brain Injury He Received in Iraq," WebMd, http://www.webmd.com/brain/features/bob-woodruff-after-traumatic-brain-injury (Accessed June 2013).

Manning, Karhy. "Blood Test for Concussions," 1 May 2013, Neuro Rehab Blog, http://neurorehabtherapy.com/bloodtest (Accessed July 2013).

Marsh, Heather. "My Discovery of Mild Traumatic Brain Injury," 16 June 11, Defence Centres for Excellence, http://www.dcoe.health.mil/blog/11-06-16/My_Discovery_of_Mild_Traumatic_Brain_Injury.aspx (Accessed June 2013).

McCloskey, Megan. "Can a Blood Test Reveal a Traumatic Brain Injury?" Stripes Central, 8 November 2011, http://www.stripes.com/blogs/stripes-central/stripes-central-1.8040/can-a-blood-test-reveal-a-traumatic-brain-injury-1.160131 (Accessed June 2013).

"Mild TBI Remains Little Understood and Hard to Diagnose," U.S. Medicine: The Voice of Federal Medicine, http://www.usmedicine.com/neurology/mild-tbi-remains-little-understood-and-hard-to-diagnose.html#.UcybrD7F1vZ , Accessed May 2013.

Mondello, Stefania, Uwe Muller, and Kevin KW Wang, "Blood-Based Diagnostics of Traumatic Brain Injuries," Expert Review of Molecular Diagnostics, January 2011 (11:1) 65-78.

Nordqvist, Joseph. "Blood Test Reveals Extent of Brain Damage Following Concussion." Medical News Today, 8 March 2013, http://www.medicalnewstoday.com/articles/257407.php (Accessed July 2013).

Pennington, Bill. "A New Way to Care for Young Brains." The New York Times, 5 May 2013. http://www.nytimes.com/2013/05/06/sports/concussion-fears-lead-to-growth-in-specialized-clinics-for-young-athletes.html?pagewanted=1&_r=2& (July 2013).

"What Are the Leading Causes of TBI?" The Centres for Disease Control, http://www.cdc.gov/traumaticbraininjury/causes.html , Accessed June 2013.

Printed in Great Britain
by Amazon